BEGINNER'S HALF-MARATHON TRAINER

W9-BPB-934

BEGINNER'S HALF-MARATHON TRAINER

THE 14-WEEK PROGRAM

TO COMPLETING A HALF-MARATHON IN YOUR BEST TIME

JON ACKLAND

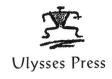

Ulysses Press

This book is dedicated to Kerri Ackland for her support, advice and patience. It is also to help her with the half-marathon she is training for.

© 2008 text Jon Ackland; programs and methodology (intellectual property) Jon Ackland Performance Lab will strongly defend any infringement

Published in the United States by
ULYSSES PRESS
P.O. Box 3440
Berkeley, CA 94703
www.ulyssespress.com

First published in New Zealand as **Compete or Complete Half Marathon** in 2006 by Random House New Zealand

ISBN10: 1-56975-636-8
ISBN13: 978-1-56975-636-2
Library of Congress Catalog Number: 2007905466

Printed in Canada by Webcom

10 9 8 7 6 5 4 3 2 1

Design: Katy Yiakmis and Amy Tansell
Layout: Amy Tansell / Words Alive
Cover design: Double R Design
Front cover photos: ©istockphoto.com
Back cover photos: ©photos.com
U.S. editorial and production: Judith Metzener, Emma Silvers, Steven Schwartz

Please note: This book has been written and published strictly for informational purposes, and in no way should be used as a substitute for consultation with health care professionals. You should not consider educational material herein to be the practice of medicine or to replace consultation with a physician or other medical practitioner. The author and publisher are providing you with information in this work so that you can have the knowledge and can choose, at your own risk, to act on that knowledge. The author and publisher also urge all readers to be aware of their health status and to consult health care professionals before beginning any health or exercise program.

CONTENTS

The origin of the half-marathon

A half-marathon is a wonderful challenge—a tremendously satisfying experience that has awesome benefits.

Before we start talking about how to train for a half-marathon, I thought I'd give you a little idea of the history you are about to run or walk into.

The history of the marathon dates back to 490 BC, when the Greeks were at war with the Persians. The Greeks won the battle and they sent an Athenian soldier, named Pheidippides, to run about 25 miles from the town of Marathon back to Athens to tell the powers-that-be that they had won. He arrived exhausted at the Athenian palace, said "Rejoice, we conquer," and promptly fell down dead. (Actually, despite the popular story, he probably didn't run from Marathon to Athens—he probably ran more like 150 miles—and he probably didn't die of exhaustion, but that ruins a good story . . . Go to *www.performancelab.co.nz* for the real story of the marathon and Pheidippides.)

The current distance for the marathon (which a half-marathon is obviously half of) was fixed at the 1908 London Olympics, at 26 miles, 385 yards. Now try working out half of that and it comes down to a pretty strange number.

So why 26 miles 385 yards? As mentioned above, the distance between Marathon and Athens is more like 25 miles. The reason it was set at the current distance was because of a queen, a king, their castle and a district in West London called Shepherd's Bush! At the 1908 Olympics, they wanted Queen Alexandra to start the event. She lived in Windsor Castle. The finishing line was White City Stadium in Shepherd's Bush. And the distance between Windsor Castle and Shepherd's Bush along the marathon course was 26 miles.

So what about the extra 385 yards? This was added so the race could finish in front of King Edward VII's Royal Box.

You are about to train for an event that originated in 490 B.C. because of a war. The first guy who did it had to run an excessively long way, and it's exactly half the distance between Windsor Castle and Shepherd's Bush.

Strange but true! Now onward and upward . . .

PART 1

Before you start

CHAPTER 1

Why do a half-marathon?

IT'S NOT REALLY ABOUT THE RUN

For thousands of years poets and philosophers have had the job of pondering the meaning of life, of wondering what life and the universe are all about. These days, more and more of us in Western cultures have the time and energy to wonder what our life is, or should be, for. Unfortunately, this can lead to "existential angst" —essentially, anxiety over our existence. People wait for life to give them meaning, or perhaps go searching for meaning, believing it's somewhere "out there."

But here is another way of thinking about the meaning of life: life will only be meaningful to you if you do (or experience) meaningful things.

Of course, what is meaningful to one person may be meaningless to another. Meaning is in the soul of the doer, which is why some people are passionate about designing clothes, others about growing roses, and still others about riding their bike. But beneath the specific attractions of fashion, gardening, and cycling, there seem to be some common themes that drive human behavior.

Achievement

Human history is a history of achievement. From Galileo to Einstein, from Amelia Earhart to Neil Armstrong, our world has been shaped by the achievements of men and women through the ages.

Humans, it seems, are not designed to sit still, either literally or metaphorically. We are constantly striving to do better—fly further, climb higher, dive deeper, run faster. Our desire to move forward energizes us, powers our creativity and, it turns out, lets us live longer.

Attitude

As we get older, it is easy to let our horizons shrink, our boundaries contract and our limitations multiply. In short, we do less, feel less, experience less.

Now, it may not surprise you to learn that a study has found that people whose lives are defined by fear and risk-avoidance tend to die younger (extreme risk-takers such as mountaineers are, of course, an exception!). Dr. Ronald Grossarth-Maticek from Heidelberg, Germany conducted a study of 10,000 people over a period of 20 years, looking at why some people live longer than others and why some people suffer less illness than others. He performed medical, physiological and psychological tests and what he concluded was that the main thing that caused people to live longer was their attitude.

Now you might be thinking, "Yeah, yeah, if I think good things, I'll live a long time." But it's not quite like that. What he discovered was that everybody has a set of limits to what they think they're capable of.

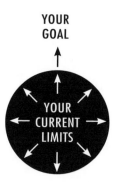

What the study found was that if you try to do something that is outside your current limits and achieve it, that expands all your horizons, all your limits, all your boundaries.

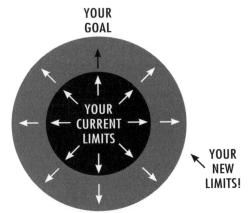

What this all means is that a lot of people who live the longest are those who keep stretching the boundaries of life, and these people also suffer the least illness. For everybody else, getting older means their world contracts, options are reduced and fewer chances are taken. If you face your fears they get smaller. If you don't face them they get bigger. It's just part of life.

In other words, your attitude plays a role in how long you live. The sooner you put up those shutters, the sooner, it seems, you will be shut off from the world—for good! So face your fears, take a few risks and keep stretching your boundaries.

When you decide to do something like a half-marathon, for a lot of you it's going to be way outside your current limits. And to go there, you have to go into the territory of fear and uncertainty. Don't let this worry you—that's what a big challenge is all about.

Self-belief

As founder of the Ford Motor Company, Henry Ford knew a few things about taking risks and being successful. He also knew a few things about people.

A great believer in goal-setting, Ford recognized that a person's attitude would determine how far a person went in life, even more than the motor car. As Ford said, "If you think you can do it, you're right; if you think you can't, you're still right."

It can be too easy to impose limits on ourselves, especially as we get older. How often have you heard someone say they can't do something because they're "too old"?

There is no denying that there are some physical realities associated with aging, but in my experience it is the "mental unrealities" that more often determine what a person will and won't do—or perhaps, more importantly, will and won't try.

As the sayings go, "Better to have played and lost, than to not have played at all" or "You miss 100% of the shots you don't take"!

Adventure

When was the last time you went on an adventure? Kids do it all the time. You can probably remember a few adventures of your own—times when you explored your boundaries by leaving the house, crossing the street, or biking to Aunty Wendy's house 12 miles away because you wanted to see if you could do it.

Steve Fossett, holder of numerous world records for ballooning, is a modern-day adventurer. Fossett is wealthy enough to sit back and live a life of leisure. But instead he chooses to live a life of adventure. Fossett takes risks—big risks—and challenges his limits, and so has experiences that almost certainly make him feel like a kid again.

So, add adventure to your life, explore your inner and outer worlds and choose to stay young.

As Australian rugby league coach Wayne Bennett says, "Don't die with the music in you."

Remember . . .
- Life's for living—chase experiences
- Challenge your limits
- Believe in yourself
- Take some (calculated) risks

Adopt a "can do" attitude and focus on success.

CHAPTER 2

Why exercise?

Simple—it's good for you! The ancient Greeks knew it. Arthur Lydiard knew it. And the modern medical community knows it.

Dr. George Sheehan (author of *Running & Being—The Total Experience*) once wrote: "Play is good for losing weight and reducing risk factors. For relieving stress and returning us to work relaxed. Play maintains our health and promotes our longevity." By "play," Sheehan meant running, swimming, cycling, dancing . . . any activity that meets our physical, emotional, and spiritual need for motion.

The road safety advertisements tell us "speed kills" but when it comes to our body, slowing to a stop can have equally disastrous results.

Quite simply, exercise is a fantastic way to help us manage our health. And if we also watch our diet, stay smoke-free, moderate our alcohol intake and get enough sleep, we can be healthier, more energetic and, yes, nicer to be around.

OK, enough of the sales pitch. Let's have a closer look at some of the ways exercise is good for us.

REDUCED RISK OF DISEASE

Researchers have been investigating the health benefits of exercise for decades. One of the best-known studies in this field is the Harvard Study. The Harvard Study looked at 50,000 people from the University of

Pennsylvania and Harvard College from 1916 through to the present day. Throughout the lives of these people, researchers tracked their medical records and collected lifestyle information. Due to the large sample size of their study they were able say that, statistically, if you do one thing lifestyle-wise, an effect is likely to happen health-wise.

What were their major findings? If you are exercising regularly you have a 31% lower risk of cancer and a 46% lower risk of heart disease. The effects are particularly pronounced for colon, breast and prostate cancers—which just happen to be the most common cancers in the Western world.

As approximately 66% of the population dies of cancer or heart disease, those findings alone would suggest you should be on your way out the door now!

The Harvard Study showed that exercise will also lower your risk of gallstones, type-2 diabetes and arthritis. And in 1970, Dr. Ralph Paffenbarger determined that if you were sedentary you were 60% more likely to get heart disease.

Better control of health risk factors

Exercise also helps us manage some of the potential contributors to disease, especially heart disease. For example, exercise can help control your cardiovascular risk factors such as cholesterol level, body weight and blood pressure. One study suggested that regular exercise would extend your expected life span by 5.7 years.

Smarter and happier

Regular exercise has been associated with a 9% increase in cognitive function (which is just a flashy way of saying you'll be smarter) and a 17% increase in happiness.

Researchers aren't precisely sure how exercise makes you happier but some possible explanations are:

- endorphins—the body's natural opiates are released into our system when we exercise, giving us a "high"
- neurotransmitters—exercise positively affects the chemicals in

the brain associated with mood control
- heat—the warmth created by exercising makes us feel good, just like spas, saunas, and hot showers seem to
- distraction—exercise distracts us from the things that make us unhappy

But whatever the reasons, people consistently report they feel better, happier, and more positive when they exercise regularly.

IMPROVED FITNESS

Regular exercise makes you more fit. How's that for stating the obvious? Of course, what you are more fit for depends on what type of exercise you do. For example, if a weightlifter wants to get more fit for weightlifting, they are generally better off lifting more weights than going swimming. In other words, we can talk about fitness or we can talk about activity, or sport-specific fitness.

When it comes to aerobic exercise such as running or walking, one area of fitness that is improved is the heart's fitness. More accurately, exercise that makes you puff improves the health of the heart and circulatory system. The other good thing about running or walking as a choice of exercise is that it makes you specifically more fit for the physical exercise you do most often—walking.

Resting heart rate fitness test

How will you know you're getting more fit? Try the following test as you move through your training program:

Measure your heart rate each morning for a couple of weeks, to establish your average resting heart rate. Take it in bed, lying down, upon waking. (Either count all your heartbeats for a minute, or count for ten seconds and multiply by six.) If you wake up to an alarm, this can raise your heart rate slightly, so rest for two to three minutes before taking it. Make allowances if you have a busy day that day (and are feeling anxious), or if you need to urinate, as both may elevate heart rate slightly. For example:

	Mon	Tue	Wed	Thu	Fri	Sat	Sun
Heart rate	76	74	75	76	74	76	77

Total heartbeats = 528, divided by seven days = 75.4. This gives you an average heart rate for the week of 75.

As you get more fit your heart will get bigger, so it will take fewer beats to do the same amount of work. Your resting heart rate will go down.

Note: If you are still tired from previous exercise, your heart rate may become elevated. If it is elevated by more than 10% of the average, have an easy day's exercise or a day off.

Aerobic exercise will not only give you a lower resting heart rate but will also enable your heart rate to return to normal more quickly after exercise. One way to assess this is to do some exercise that elevates your heart rate, recover for 3 minutes, then see what your heart rate has dropped to.

BOOSTED IMMUNE SYSTEM

Research has shown that moderate levels of exercise improve your immune system, making you less likely to catch colds, for example, and more likely to recover quickly when you do.

Studies show that people who walk regularly have half the number of sick days of their sedentary counterparts (5.1 days compared with 10.8 days through the winter). In a 1989 *Runner's World* survey, 61% of the 700 respondents were less sick. In another survey, 90% of experienced runners also experienced the same good health. (Of course, too much exercise—or stress—can compromise the immune system. We are much more likely to pick up bugs when we are exhausted or under pressure for long periods of time.)

The lymphatic system is a key player in helping the body battle infections. But to do its job the system needs to move lymph, a fluid containing white blood cells, around the body.

While the cardiac system has the heart as its pump, the lymphatic system relies on the movement of muscles to transport lymph to the places it needs to go, and to remove the biochemical waste and bacteria we want to dispose of. Running and walking are great ways to help the lymphatic system do its job well.

IMPROVED FUNCTIONALITY

Exercise also improves our functionality. In life, what happens is you're born, you lie on your back and you drool, and you look at the ceiling. Then, when you reach the age of about 20 to 30 you are at your peak of physical functionality. Then you have a choice. You either choose to maintain your functional levels, you follow the "most people" path, or you just don't care. This affects what happens over the following years.

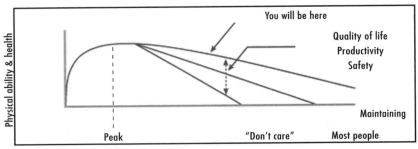

If you choose to exercise and pay attention to your health you'll maintain your functionality—the whole "use it or lose it" mentality—you'll stay up on the top line in the above graphic. Your quality of life is going to be greater and your productivity in later life is going to be greater.

The middle line is how most people age. The lowest line is the "don't care" line—the people who don't pay attention to their health at all, and who therefore age faster than average. There is a very good reason why some people look young or old for their age!

In one sense, our loss of functionality is what we call "aging." Of course, we can't stop ourselves getting older, but we can at the very least slow down the so-called "aging process." How? By keeping active—physically and mentally.

If you want to keep up with your kids and grandkids, the message is simple: keep moving, and keep learning.

Chronological vs. biological aging

In Dr. Michael Roizen's book *Real Age,* he describes the difference between chronological aging and biological aging. Chronological aging is aging in years. Biological aging is aging in terms of life processes. There's a big difference.

If you take three cars built in the year 2000 (same model, same make), and you leave one in the garage and never drive it; you take another one and go out and thrash it; and you take the third one and drive it as it was designed to be driven, which car is going to be in the best shape by 2007?

Well, the first car's engine has seized and the second has blown up . . . but the third engine is functioning fine. The cars are the same chronological age, but totally different mechanical (biological) ages.

Dr. Roizen looked at literally thousands of research articles and was able to establish the difference between the average mortality rate and the mortality rate based on a particular lifestyle trait.

To give an exercise example, if you are 35 years of age, male, and you exercise, your biological age is 31. If you are 55 years of age, female, and exercise, your biological age is 52.

Reducing your body fat (gauged using the body mass index or BMI), blood pressure and cholesterol can also take years off your chronological age: up to 4.5 years to be precise. A 35-year-old male could potentially end up 26.9 and a 55-year-old could potentially be 47.5 years young. You choose!

Conversely, Roizen found that if you smoke cigarettes, there is on average a three-year reduction in your life expectancy.

By the way, if you have more than 300 orgasms a year, your biological age is three years less than your chronological age. And if you have a dog, you can be six months younger biologically as well. (These two statistics are not, we hope, associated.)

It's biological aging which is most important. In other words, you are only as old as you feel!

SENSE OF ACHIEVEMENT

Other "aging" research looks at the relationship between self-esteem and longevity. People with higher levels of self-esteem tend to age better. I guess it's about the thoughts and emotions your body is bathed in day after day. You need to be able to look back and say, "2002 was good because . . . ; 2003 was good because . . . ; 2004 was good because . . ."

It's about making every year count, every year an experience, every year an adventure. When you get to 105 and you're on your deathbed, you can look back over your life and say, "Wow—boy, did I live it!"

Ask yourself, "When I get to 105 years old and look back on my life . . . what will I see?"

Other positive effects of running or walking
- Muscle tone will increase in your legs
- Muscle endurance goes up
- The ligaments and tendons in your legs get stronger, which means less chance of injuries while active in other areas
- Bone density remains high as you age (very important for postmenopausal women)
- Exercise keeps you more productive in a work environment
- Improved quality of life
- Increased self-esteem

You go out, take it easy, train and chat with a friend, and you get all these benefits without even trying!

A REAL-LIFE EXAMPLE

Here is the physiological data on the staff of two multinational companies training to prepare for a half-marathon over approximately 14 weeks.

Company 1
Aerobic Fitness
Before 38.07 ml/kg/min
After   46.63 ml/kg/min
Change 8.56 ml/kg/min (22% improvement)

Cholesterol
Before   4.45 mmol/L
After   4.23 mmol/L
Change   4.9%

Average body weight
Before   185 lbs.
After   176 lbs.
Change   9 lbs.
550 participants lost a total of 4835 lbs.

Average heart rate after three minutes' rest from exercise
Before   100 beats per minute
After   89 beats per minute
Change   11 beats per minute

General
- 87% of participants felt better/more motivated after the event
- Fitness levels went from average to very fit when compared with the general population
- Cholesterol went from good to very good
- The average weight-loss was 9 lbs. and the maximum weight-loss, when combined with good nutrition, 62 lbs. The 550 participants lost more than 2 tons of fat between them!

Company 2

In Company 2, 73% of participants were novice or recreational runners, and 20% had never exercised before. After the completion of the program:

68%	had higher energy levels
76%	felt healthier
90%	felt more fit
96%	wanted to do something similar again
92%	felt the program had an impact on their overall health
46%	had lost weight (140 people lost a total of 487 lbs.)
85%	were more motivated
89%	completed the training program (most of the 11% who didn't complete was due to injury)
99%	completed the event.

CHAPTER 3

How do I know you can do this?

Let's deal with a myth first. You have no doubt heard the phrase "No pain, no gain." Well, for beginners this is not the best way to approach training. If I cut my hand with a knife I experience extreme pain. That's my body's way of saying, "Well, that was really dumb." If I stick my hand on a hot element and fry it, apart from the bad smell, I experience extreme pain. Again, my body says, "Really dumb!"

If you come back into the house from a training run dragging one leg and bleeding from the ears, and you can work out your pulse rate by watching your purple face throb in the mirror, then you've got a serious problem.

In sports, like in life, the "no pain, no gain" thing is a load of garbage. Pain is a sign you've done something dumb! Or, more specifically, if you experience pain when you are training, something is wrong.

When you are new to a sport or exercise, it's not about pain. It's about taking it nice and easy and working your way into it.

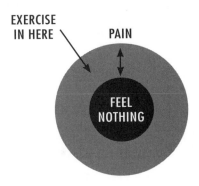

23

Your first workout might be just ten minutes long. You might be thinking: "It's not even worth putting my shoes on for ten minutes." But ten minutes soon becomes 20, and 20 becomes 30, and 30 becomes 40, and 40 becomes 60, and yes, 60 becomes 90.

Before you know it you can do a half-marathon. That's how we work it. We want your fitness to sneak up on you. We don't want training to be a painful chore. That's not smart training.

TRUST ME ON THIS

Most of the people I've worked with who are new to running are surprised at what they are able to achieve. They are also surprised at how easy it was to reach a goal they may not have thought possible just a few months earlier.

Interestingly, most people who do not complete the training program are not beginners. They are people who have some experience. How come? Well, the beginners start out nice and easy, while the more experienced people tend to go too fast, too soon and get injured.

The lesson? In the first month of training take it really, really easy—no matter how much or how little experience you have. That way you give yourself the best chance of getting to the starting line healthy and smiling. And once you're there? Well, the completion rate for people who have followed our programs has been as high as 99%.

WHAT DO YOU WANT TO ACHIEVE?

As I pointed out earlier, studies have highlighted two factors that limit what people achieve: fear and lack of belief. People find it hard to believe that they can do some things. And they are scared to take a risk, scared to try something new.

Of course, we're all limited to some extent by what we believe we can do and by our fear of failure. Here is a quote which might give you the courage to challenge the limits you put on yourself:

If you think you are beaten, you are. If you think you dare not, you don't. If you'd like to win but you think you can't, it's almost certain you won't.

If you think you'll lose, you're lost, for out in this world we find success begins with a person's belief. It's all a state of mind. If you think you're outclassed, you are. You've got to think high to rise. You've got to be sure of yourself before you can ever win a prize. Life's battles don't always go to the stronger or faster one, but sooner or later the one who wins is the one who thinks they can.

And now here's a little quote about taking risks:

To laugh is to risk appearing a fool. To weep is to risk being called sentimental. To reach out to another is to risk showing your true self. To place your ideas and dreams before a crowd is to risk being called naive. To love is to risk not being loved in return. To live is to risk dying. To hope is to risk despair. To try is to risk failure. The greatest risk in life is to risk nothing. The person who risks nothing does nothing, has nothing, is nothing and becomes nothing. Only the person who risks is truly free.

A lot of you will be thinking: "Do I really want to try this?" or, "I don't even know if I can do it." That's normal. When facing a task that challenges our perception of what we can do, we will have doubts.

The trick is to understand that everyone who has achieved anything worthwhile has had doubts. But they found the courage and the energy to start anyway. And once they started down their path to achievement, they found those doubts started to disappear (slowly at first) and lose their power. And then, miraculously, those doubts gave way to visions of success!

THE TRAINING TIME REQUIREMENT

So, who can do this event? Almost anybody who is prepared to check boxes, do a little bit of training and take a risk.

There are 168 hours in a week. The maximum training time per week for most of you will be four hours (two or three workouts) and even this won't need to happen for some period of time. Your minimum training requirement might only be 40 minutes for the entire week to start with! Therefore, for most of you the maximum time requirement is 1.5 to 2% of the whole week. If you want to race, you will need around six to eight hours (five or six workouts) per week.

Still, you might say, "I don't have time for this." In fact, 50% of people say that in this situation. But remember, we've talked about what exercise does to your biological age. You'll probably live longer, so therefore you actually have *more* time to do this!

What do you get for your time and effort?

Well, the first thing is that you'll push back your boundaries. You'll have a young attitude; you'll be younger mentally. You'll probably live longer because of it.

Secondly, the Harvard Study says you'll age more slowly, you'll be younger for your years. You'll be young physically. And furthermore, you'll have a huge improvement in your health profile. You'll have 31% less risk of cancer, 43% less risk of heart disease. That is *huge*.

Further to that, real-life examples show that this is not a con. We know it works.

The numerous studies on achievement say that most people self-limit. You won't. You will experience *everything*. You get to have an adventure.

And all of this will be for 1.5% of your time.

You might think, "This guy is doing a sales pitch on me!" *Of course I am* . . . but everything I have covered is true. It's just that most people don't know this stuff, and knowing it helps to make you and I want to exercise.

People often say, "Why would you want to exercise?" Knowing what I know and hopefully knowing what you now know, your answer would be, "*Why wouldn't you?*"

You have two choices: you can sit on the couch and watch the world go by, or you can get off the couch and *be* the world going by!

I know who I'd rather be!

CHAPTER 4

A few ideas for all the gear

You may need to make a few small investments before you start training. Running in bare feet is not that much fun. A lot of beginners may feel intimidated by all this, but you don't want—or need—to dress up like an Olympic marathon champion. There is, however, a reason why they have all the gear: it's comfortable and it works.

SHOES

Depending on your running speed and technique, your shoes take a load of two to five times your body weight per stride. At a standard speed and at three times their body weight, a 154 lb. runner's shoes experience a stride load of 463 lbs.! Good shoes are important to look after you and your feet.

It is vitally important that you have a good pair of walking or running shoes. If you don't, here's how to choose the right ones.

Step 1: What are you?

The wet foot test:
Step in some water and then stand on a flat, dry area of ground. See which of the following illustrations your footprints look most like.

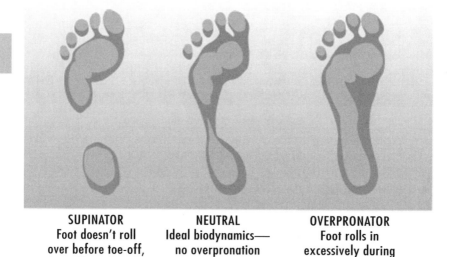

SUPINATOR	NEUTRAL	OVERPRONATOR
Foot doesn't roll over before toe-off, but rolls to the side	Ideal biodynamics— no overpronation	Foot rolls in excessively during the foot strike

The running/walking test:
Ask someone to watch you running or walking from behind. Compare what they see with the illustration below to confirm the wet foot test.

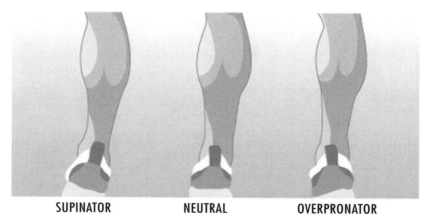

SUPINATOR	NEUTRAL	OVERPRONATOR

These two tests allow you to initially place yourself into one of three running categories. You're either:

- a *supinator*—your foot doesn't roll inward before toe touches, but rolls to the side
- *neutral*—ideal: no overpronation
- an *overpronator*—your foot rolls excessively inward during the foot strike.

The reason for this initial categorization is that shoe manufacturers make shoes for these three types of running or walking gait. Once you have been categorized, this eliminates two-thirds of the shoes available on the market.

If this is a bit of a pain, go to a sports-shoe store that analyzes how you walk or run. Don't feel intimidated: lots of people like you get this done every day. You are not the odd one out.

Once you have found the category you fit into—supinator, neutral or overpronator—apply the following tests at your local shoe store.

Step 2: Dealing with both feet

Foot folding line:
This is the line or crease that the front of the shoe folds along. This line should coincide with the ball of your foot. If you have long or short toes, the folding line can be too far forward or too far back, interfering with your running or walking gait and possibly creating a greater chance of injury or "hot spots."

Hold the shoe horizontally and longitudinally and push your hands slightly together and you will see the fold line. Measure from the line to the tip of the shoe. Compare this to the length of your foot from the center of the ball of the foot to the tip of the big toe. They should match.

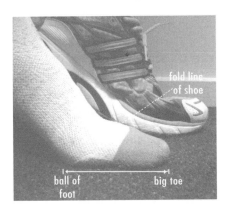

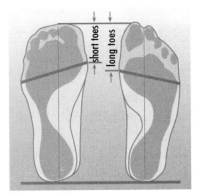

SHORT TOES
Shoe fold line needs to be further forward

LONG TOES
Shoe fold line needs to be further back

Some shoes have such a rigid sole that they don't bend easily along a fold line at all. These should be avoided.

Shoe length:
Watch shoe sizing as it is notoriously different between brands. To find the correct length, take out the insole and place your foot on it. There should be about a thumb-width or a half-inch of room at the end of the longest toe. This is so the foot can slide forward as it unwinds during running or walking.

It is better to try on new shoes in the afternoon, as your feet are usually bigger than in the morning.

The following graphics show why a half-inch of room between your toes and the end of your shoe is important during a running or walking motion:

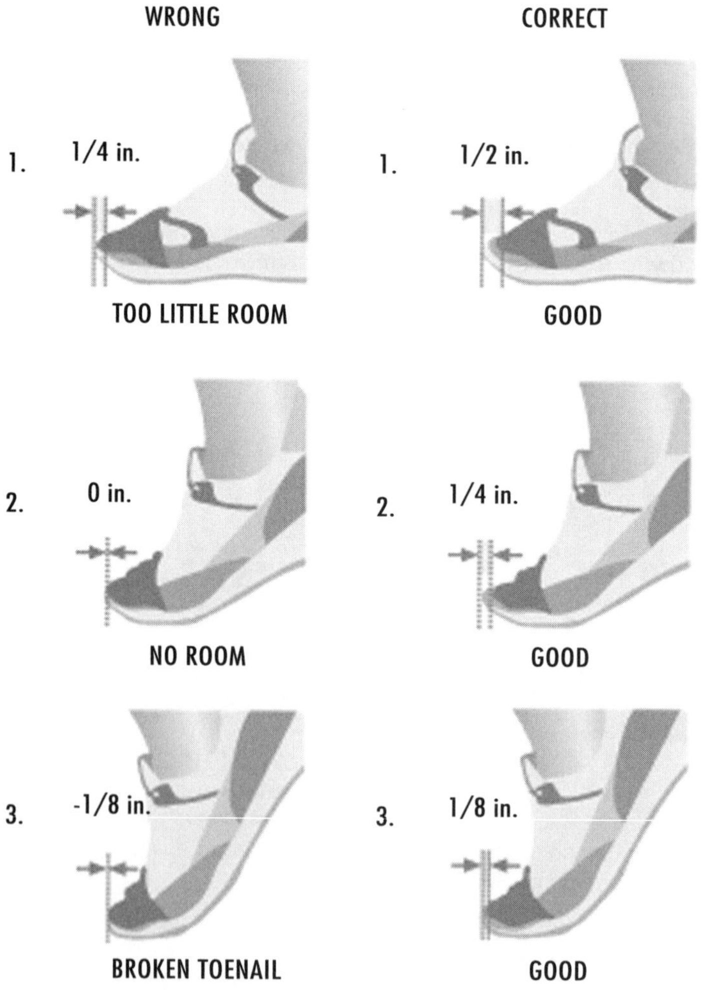

WRONG	CORRECT
1. 1/4 in.	1. 1/2 in.
TOO LITTLE ROOM	GOOD
2. 0 in.	2. 1/4 in.
NO ROOM	GOOD
3. -1/8 in.	3. 1/8 in.
BROKEN TOENAIL	GOOD

Shoe width:
Very few manufacturers make different shoe widths. Therefore the only way to be sure the width is correct is to try the shoes on. Be aware of the level of side pressure through the ball of the foot when walking and running. This should feel comfortable.

Step 3: Heels and ankles

Heel position and support:
Put your foot in the shoe and tie the laces. Put one foot behind the other and place the toe of the rear shoe against the heel of the front shoe to hold it on the ground. Now try to lift your foot out of the front shoe. This should be difficult.

Also check the seam down the inside middle of the shoe heel. This can be quite prominent in some shoes and can cause blistering and chafing. There should be no up and down movement of the shoe against your heel when you walk.

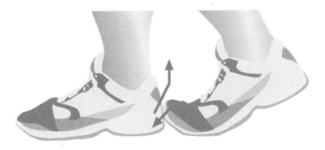

Ankle freedom:
The gap between the bottom of your ankle joint and the rim of the shoe directly below should be at least 1/8 of an inch. If the rim is too high for the ankle, it can cause blistering and chafing after a few miles of running or walking.

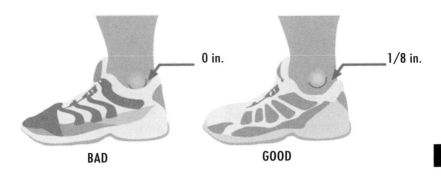

0 in.   1/8 in.

BAD   GOOD

Step 4: A little lace and a few tricks

Lacing:

There are various lacing methods but the key is to ensure that you have good control of your foot, and that it will contact and roll properly.

It's good to think of your lacing in two parts: front of the shoe and foot arch area. Lacing over the front of the shoe can often be a little less tight to ensure the foot is not too squashed, but the foot arch area needs to be a little tighter. Your toes shouldn't slide back and forward but your foot can relax a little bit.

Other notes on shoes:

- Try to test-drive shoes before you buy
- If you have abnormally narrow or wide feet, make this a consideration
- Do not compromise fit for cost
- Break in new shoes slowly by alternating them with your old pairs
- If you have found a shoe you like, stick to it
- Pretty colors and designs don't help you to run or walk better
- Bigger people require more support in a shoe

SOCKS

Buy breathable socks to wick sweat away from your foot. Look for materials such as ClimaCool, CoolMax or other synthetics designed to do this. It is worth spending the extra money to get good socks, otherwise your feet will sweat and you are more likely to get blisters.

CLOTHING

Key aspects of running clothing are:

- Color—no, I don't mean how pretty it looks. Lighter-colored clothing will tend to reflect sunlight and therefore heat, which may keep you cooler.
- Breathability—buy clothing that wicks sweat away from the skin and allows it to evaporate on the surface of the garment (e.g. clothing made with material such as ClimaCool). This will keep you cooler when it's hot and warmer when it's cold.
- Fit—try to get loose-fitting clothing, which helps air to circulate

and is therefore better for controlling your body temperature.
- Cap/visor—light-colored, breathable hats that are not too tight-fitting are best.

CHAFING

Wearing long cycle-type shorts, either on their own or under running shorts, helps if you get chafing between the thighs. You can also wear tracksuit pants, although they can feel a little hot in the summer. You can also apply Vaseline to areas that chafe, such as the inside of thighs and backs of the armpits. In cold weather it is often useful for men to put Vaseline or Band-Aids over their nipples, since these can chafe and cause serious discomfort. Women usually wear sports bras so this is not a factor for them.

PART 2

How to train

CHAPTER 5

Show me the training!

The first thing we have to do is define what "training" actually is. *Training is showing your body what happens on the day of the event.* Another way to describe training is to say it's like charades. You can't talk to your body and tell it what is going to happen and what you want it to do; this gets you sent off for various psychiatric tests. What you have to do is take your body and *show* it the actions it will be required to do on the day.

By the time you get to the event, your body, through the actions you have shown it, should know the technique, the distance, the terrain, the weather, the course, how to use the aid stations and the speed at which you intend to do the event—be it to complete or compete for a winning medal. You will have practiced all this in training.

In its simplest form, this is all training is. If your body is prepared for everything that will happen on the day of your half-marathon, you will have a fantastic day. You just need a plan that incorporates all these points at the correct times to help you maximize the time and effort you put in. You need a *smart* training plan.

A training plan is a way of organizing your effort and time into the most effective workouts so that you get the best result for what you put in. It is a way of organizing a bunch of good ideas on how to get fit and strong into some sort of manageable order so that what you do is as effective as possible.

But before we fully get into the training plan, we need to see what the plan is made up of.

Note: Because this book contains programs for walkers and runners—and walk-runners—often we will use the term "run" when describing a workout. If you are preparing to walk a half-marathon, please read this as "walk" where appropriate.

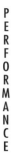

Part 2

THE IMPORTANCE OF RECOVERY

When learning about training, almost everyone initially misses out on getting to know the poor cousin of training—*recovery*—which is just as important, just not as obvious. To tell you about how to "train smart," I have to show you how training makes you more fit. So let's start with how improving your physical performance works.

Let's set the scene . . . It's 10,000 years ago and you are wandering down some track in your designer leopard-skin with your club over your shoulder and a bad haircut. A saber-tooth tiger jumps out from behind a rock and chases you. You run as fast as you can, manage to get away and hide in a cave.

While your mind is saying, "That was close!" your body's saying, "Yeah, too close! Next time I'm going to run faster." And so your body adapts by increasing its capacity to escape big cats with attitudes.

This is not rocket science. Or even animal science. But the underlying principle is important. *Your body adapts specifically to a stimulus you place on it to improve.* It's a physiological survival mechanism. Here's how it works.

After you exercise, your body gets tired. If you exercised for, say, 30 minutes, your performance would drop compared to when you started (see B in the graph below).

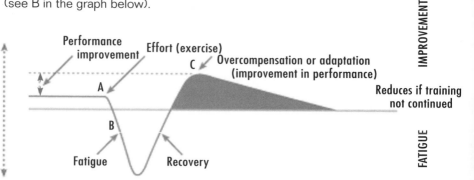

If you rested long enough to recover, your body would respond by preparing itself for another bout of exercise. This makes sense. But the clever part is the way the body responds.

Your body *overcompensates* for the stress (training) you exposed it to, so that next time that stress or training comes along, it can cope more easily (see C in the graph on the previous page). That is how we get more fit.

Part 2

I bet you're saying, "Yeah, that's obvious." Think about this, though . . .

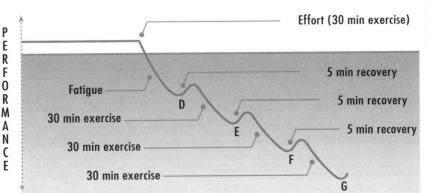

If you did 30 minutes of training, you would get tired (see D in the graph above). If you then had five minutes of recovery, had a cup of coffee and a cookie, and did another 30 minutes of training, you'd get more tired. And your performance would go down (see E in the graph above).

If you then had five minutes of recovery, another cup of coffee and another cookie, then did another 30 minutes of training, you'd be even more tired. And your performance would go down even further (see F in the graph above).

And, at the risk of being boring, if you had another five minutes of recovery, another cup of coffee and let's make it a chocolate this time, then another 30 minutes of training, you'd be even more tired. And your performance would go down even further (see G in the graph above).

The pattern is clear. Every time you train, you get tired and your performance gets worse.

This is critical to understanding how you exercise — but it seems backward, doesn't it? You think, "When I train I will get more fit." Not true!

When you train you get worse (more tired). It's when you *recover* from training that you get more fit. The recovery part is just as important as the training part.

If you don't recover, you don't get any better. And you will probably get worse.

People often say to me, "I'm going to go out and do my training even if I'm really tired, because I feel guilty if I don't." Knowing what I know about training and recovery, I'd feel guilty if I went out and trained in that condition!

The training/recovery balance is all important—never train more than you can recover from. You always want to go out the door and get a return for your efforts, otherwise it's a waste of time.

Now, let's look at the flip side of the training/recovery story. If you went out and did 20 minutes of exercise, then let your body recover and adapt, you would achieve a certain level of fitness (see C in the graph below).

If the next time you went out you did 25 minutes of exercise, your body would adapt to a higher level (see D in the graph below). If the next time you went out you did 30 minutes, your body would then, as long as you recovered, adapt to an even higher level (see E in the graph below). Almost before you are even aware of it, you can run a half-marathon!

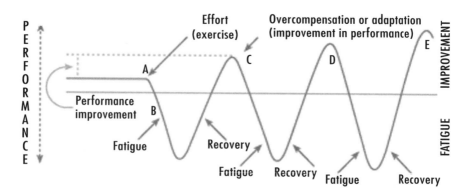

This is how training should work. This is how you improve. Therefore, it is essential that your training program has strategies for recovery, so you're constantly getting maximum return for the time you spend training. You train and then recover to "absorb" the training. Keep it smart! Don't waste time and energy!

CHAPTER 6

Adapting and maintaining

Let's now set another scene . . .

It's 6: 30 p.m. and you're off for your usual 30-minute run on the same course at the same intensity. You have been doing this for three months now and you really want to get fit for the half-marathon that is coming up. You do 30 minutes of running or walking three times a week, each and every week. So how are you going? How much improvement are you getting?

The simple answer is *none*. If you train the same way every time, what your body says is, "Great, I don't have to do anything new. So I'll stay the same."

This is important for two reasons.

First, it highlights the need to *keep changing the training stimulus*. Your body will not adapt unless it has something to adapt to.

Second, it highlights the need for *progression*.

Some people think, "I don't need to start with small amounts of training, I'll just get into the big distances right away and I'll do big distances week after week after week after week." But as suggested above, there's a problem with that. If you build your training up too quickly you do get improvement, but if you then do the same distance week after week, you soon start to plateau, and you get little improvement from that point onwards.

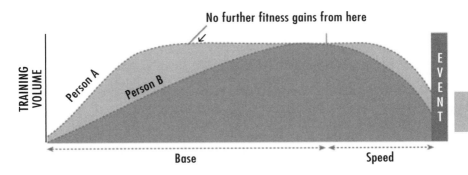

No further fitness gains from here

At this point *you're not training, you're maintaining.* If you're 75 years old and you want to keep yourself healthy, then maintain. If you want to improve your performance or prepare for a half-marathon, you need to train.

Of course, you also start off with such small training volumes because you don't want to get injured. But equally, you don't want high distances too early as you will soon be maintaining, not training. And that's not smart.

As the above graph shows, Person B does less training than Person A, particularly early in the program, but both reach the same peak volume and Person B will be fresher for the event.

RECOVERY STRATEGIES—BALANCING TRAINING WITH REST

When you look at the training programs on pages 56 to 67, you will see they have "build" and "recover" across the top of the training volume totals. This means you have building weeks, where you're doing lots of training, and recovery weeks where you train less and your body is given an opportunity to absorb the training you've been doing.

Weekly recovery

If you build your training for a few weeks and then drop the amount of training down a little so you can recover from the mild cumulative fatigue, you will be able to "absorb" the training you have done. You can then start to increase your training again and get returns on the effort.

If you continue to "push out" bigger and bigger training volumes week after week, at some point soon you begin to lose the return on your training because you are too tired or injured or ill to "absorb" the training.

This means you need a recovery strategy where you have building weeks and recovery weeks. You get more improvement for less training—kind of cool, really.

There will be harder *building weeks* where you train more, do hills, do some speed work or increase your training distance, and easier *recovery weeks* to rest from the harder weeks and allow you to have a life.

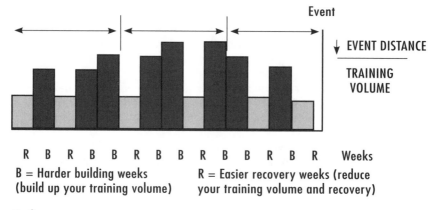

R B R B B R B B R B B R B R   Weeks

B = Harder building weeks (build up your training volume)

R = Easier recovery weeks (reduce your training volume and recovery)

Daily recovery

This building/recovery strategy across the weeks is also repeated within the weeks. Indeed, the whole program is set up to ensure that you recover adequately, so that your body absorbs the maximum amount of training that you do, and therefore you get maximum return for the time you spend training (see graphic on page 45).

Three key rules of training are:
- balance
- balance
- balance.

The training programs in this book are designed to make sure "like" workouts are kept away from each other. If you keep long workouts away from long workouts, hills away from hills and speed away from speed, this means more recovery between "like" workouts and therefore more improvement.

The psychotic example ("I don't have anything else in my life except running and need psychological counseling"):

Mon	Tue	Wed	Thu	Fri	Sat	Sun
Easy	Speed/Hills	Easy	Long	Day off	Speed/Hills	Long

The "I've got a life outside of running" example—for those who have friends/family:

Mon	Tue	Wed	Thu	Fri	Sat	Sun
Day off	Speed/Hills	Day off	Long	Day off	Speed/Hills	Long

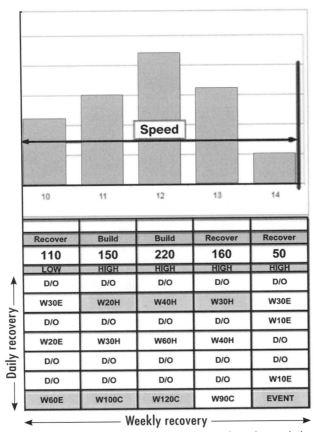

	Recover	Build	Build	Recover	Recover
	110	**150**	**220**	**160**	**50**
	LOW	HIGH	HIGH	HIGH	HIGH
	D/O	D/O	D/O	D/O	D/O
	W30E	W20H	W40H	W30H	W30E
	D/O	D/O	D/O	D/O	W10E
	W20E	W30H	W60H	W40H	D/O
	D/O	D/O	D/O	D/O	D/O
	D/O	D/O	D/O	D/O	W10E
	W60E	W100C	W120C	W90C	EVENT

So in the programs we have weekly recovery and we have daily recovery that allows you to balance training with rest. This maximizes your return and minimizes the time and effort you need to put in.

CHAPTER 7

The "Three Amigos"

OK, now that you know how training works, it's time to introduce you to the "Three Amigos."

The "Three Amigos" —The three basic workouts

There are three main workouts:

Long

Long workouts improve your endurance and allow you to do the distance of the event. You need to build up to close to the race distance two to six weeks before the event, depending on your fitness (the more fit you are, the longer build-up you can have, e.g. beginners will reach this point with only two weeks to go). You will find that this has been incorporated into your program.

Hills

Hill training is conducted to increase your strength and ability to sustain energy during the event. It's your legs that "go" first in a half-marathon so hill work is very important to improve this.

Hill training is usually conducted at an easy pace. You can do faster-pace hill efforts but in most cases easy hill running will suffice. In fact, most people do their hill training too hard.

Often a runner or walker will not reduce their stride length as they go up a hill, and feel that they need to "work it" up the hill. Consequently they exhaust themselves and end up disliking hills and not being able to do as many hills in the workout.

The idea is that when you do the half-marathon, some of your speed will come from pushing only slightly harder with your legs than you usually do when you train. It is not a huge difference in muscular effort. Therefore your training should mirror this. Running or walking up a hill will load the muscles of your legs anyway, so this is all that is required.

Look to run or walk up hills by shortening your stride and keeping your leg turnover up: taking "baby steps." Remember that your legs only need to be a little more loaded than when you are running on the flat terrain. Don't try to push up the hills; aim to run more hills rather than do them harder.

As you get closer to the event, move from more hilly runs to more rolling hills such as you would find on a golf course. Watch out for the golf balls though!

Try to do a lot of your hill work on grass or trails, since downhill running creates a lot of impact on the legs and concrete is not very forgiving. Also, as you tire your feet may start to splay outwards like a duck as you go up the hills; try to keep your toes pointed forward in this situation to avoid groin strains.

Speed

Speed work improves your ability to get used to "racing" and improves your speed. It is an optional extra. If you want to simply complete or walk the event, speed work may not be a factor in your training. However, if you want to compete, you've got to go faster in order to go faster.

Speed work involves introducing your body to small amounts of race-pace effort for initially short periods of time, leading up to slightly longer periods as you get closer to the event.

Your body cannot tolerate too much of this type of training, so try to be conservative with your speed efforts. The training programs usually involve short periods at race pace—such as five minutes—within the total workout, and occasionally time trials. These short training efforts, known as intervals, get the body conditioned. Then more experienced athletes can move on to several time trials.

As I said earlier, training is showing your body what will happen on the day of the event so speed work should be "snippets" of this. When doing speed work don't overwork yourself: show your body the intensity that you think it will experience on the day—no more. *Harder is not better.* You may find other situations in which "it hurts so it must be good" makes sense, but none apply to a first-timer's half-marathon performance.

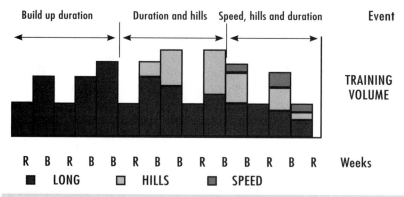

To put it all together, you have the "Three Amigos"—long, hills and speed—and you have balance, where you adapt between bouts of "like" training. The order of training moves from technique to building up your running or walking distances so you know you can complete the duration, then building up your strength, and finally building up your ability to endure the speed.

Put simply, all training is built on these small but fundamental principles. It is all controlled by the training program. The program ensures that every time you train you get the maximum return on your time and effort—and that's smart training.

BEFORE AND AFTER THE "THREE AMIGOS"

Warm-ups

A warm-up is your way of telling your body that you are about to exercise and what you will do in the workout. Start gently and build into it, showing your body several short bursts of the intensity that you will perform at if necessary. The higher the intensity of a workout, the longer the warm-up should be; for instance, 15 to 20 minutes for intervals, 20 to 30 minutes for races.

Breaking out in a sweat means that your warm-up is satisfactory, because it indicates that you have raised your body's internal temperature.

For almost all of your training:
To warm up for almost all of your training you just want to start slowly into the workout for the first five or ten minutes, since you will be exercising at a comfortable pace.

For speed work:
If you don't warm up and you have to do six intervals as part of your workout, it will take you the first two intervals to fully warm up. It means that only four intervals were worthwhile; the first two were useless.

If you are supposed to do six and you only do four good ones, you might as well save time and energy by doing a good warm-up and just doing four intervals. Train smart—don't waste time and effort.

Stretching:
The traditional recommendation is that you do your warm-up, stretch and then move into the workout. While this is true in principle, you will find that this is rare among runners and walkers in practice. For most people, it is probably fine just to start into the training gently. If you have been desk-bound in the same position all day then it is advisable to stretch, however.

If you are stretching, here is how you do it. Each stretch should be performed in a slow, controlled manner. Move slowly into the stretch until you feel the first sensation of a stretch—any more tension can cause overstretching, which results in muscle tightening rather than loosening.

You should not bounce during the stretch, and no sudden, jerky movements are advised; both can cause injury. Hold each stretch for ten to 30 seconds (any less is not really beneficial) and try to fully relax the muscle being stretched, and the surrounding muscles.

Be sensitive to tension in the muscle, since this will determine how many repetitions of the stretch you should perform. This also acts as a guide to improvement in your stretching and prevents overstretching.

Note that more stretching and a longer warm-up will be required if you train in the morning, because you will generally be less flexible at this time of the day.

A SELECTION OF STRETCHES

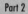
Part 2

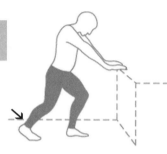

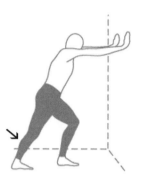

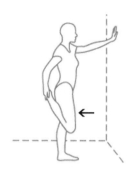

**LOWER LEG—
SHORT CALF STRETCH**

**LOWER LEG—
LONG CALF STRETCH**

**UPPER LEG —
QUADRICEPS**

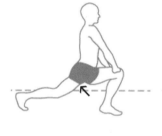

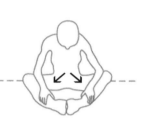

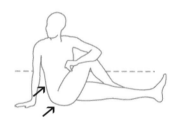

HIP FLEXORS

INNER THIGH/GROIN

**LOWER BACK AND
BUTTOCKS**

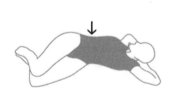

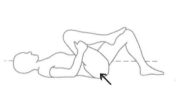

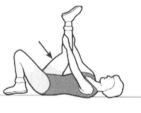

LOWER BACK

BUTTOCKS

HAMSTRINGS

Cool-downs

A cool-down is where you allow the body to clear all the waste products that accumulate during exercise. Why bother? If you clear out the "junk" you recover quicker. Why is this important? The quality of your next workout will be better and you'll feel better for the rest of the day after the workout, instead of feeling tired, with leaden muscles. Slow down in the last five minutes of your workout and relax a little.

Stretching:
Stretching after exercise is where you make most of your flexibility gains. It is often very good to go home and stretch in front of the TV while you catch up on the day's news—it's more relaxing than doing your stretches immediately after the workout when you are tired and maybe less comfortable.

For lazy stretchers:
Some athletes do not like stretching. If you are one of those athletes, at least try to stretch up to three times per week rather than not at all (it might help to think about which you hate more: stretching or injuries!). It's best in this case to stretch before and after, or at least after, your shorter workouts, when you have more time and are less tired.

Stretching is always more important in the cool-down than in the warm-up. If you decide to stretch only during cool-down, do a longer exercise warm-up before starting your workout.

Carbo-up:

If you eat carbohydrates within 60 to 120 minutes of completing your workout, your body will recover much faster than if you don't (and it'll love you for it!). In the first hour after exercise the body is in an energy-depleted state and, if provided with carbohydrates, it will super-compensate for the loss of energy due to the workout, absorbing more energy from them.

CHAPTER 8

Choosing a training program

We've talked about it, now it's time for you to select your training program. First you need to work out what event you are going to do, and how far away it is.

My goal event is: . . . .

Make sure it's far enough away to train for properly, but not so far away that you get bored. An event nine to 16 weeks away is the ideal range to look at. The programs in this book are all 14 weeks long.

Now you need to find the program that matches your goals and your level of fitness and ability.

Do you want to walk the event?	Use program 1 (pages 56–57)
Do you want to walk/run the event?	Use program 2 (pages 58–59)
Do you want to run the event, but are an absolute beginner, starting from scratch?	Use program 3 (pages 60–61)
Do you want to run the event and have some running experience, even if you've never done an event like this before?	Use program 4 (pages 62–63)
Do you want to run the event for a competitive time?	Use program 5 (pages 64–65)

Have you run a half-marathon before and want to "race" the event, working on improving your speed? Use program 6 (pages 66–67)

You can also contact Performance Lab direct to discuss personalized training options, at info@performancelab.co.nz, or check out *www.performancelab.co.nz*.

Part 2

UNDERSTANDING HOW YOUR TRAINING PROGRAM WORKS

Let's take a closer look at the training program you have chosen. It will look something like this example. It might look a little complex to start with, but we'll go through it and you'll find it's actually quite simple.

Along the top of the training program, below the graph, you have the number of weeks in the program and the total volume of training for each week. Down the left side you have the days of the week. Therefore, if you were exercising on Thursday in the third week (see area highlighted in grey), you'd be doing a 20-minute workout.

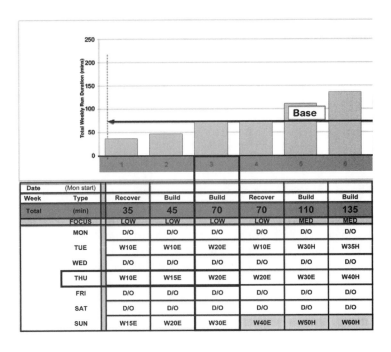

Date	(Mon start)						
Week	Type	Recover	Build	Build	Recover	Build	Build
Total	(min)	35	45	70	70	110	135
	FOCUS	LOW	LOW	LOW	LOW	MED	MED
	MON	D/O	D/O	D/O	D/O	D/O	D/O
	TUE	W10E	W10E	W20E	W10E	W30H	W35H
	WED	D/O	D/O	D/O	D/O	D/O	D/O
	THU	W10E	W15E	W20E	W20E	W30E	W40H
	FRI	D/O	D/O	D/O	D/O	D/O	D/O
	SAT	D/O	D/O	D/O	D/O	D/O	D/O
	SUN	W15E	W20E	W30E	W40E	W50H	W60H

Going into more detail, the numbers represent the number of minutes of each workout. For example, 20 means a 20-minute workout.

E means *easy running or walking*. Easy means easy conversation pace. So if you are running or walking along and you are talking about something and going "talk, talk, talk . . . GASP . . . talk, talk, talk . . . GASP . . ." then you've probably got it a little bit wrong. You should be able to have a conversation for the entire time.

For those on walking programs, W means *walk*. RW means *run some, walk some*. Start by running from one lamppost to the next. Walk until you are ready to run again. Move up to running two lampposts, then three, and so on.

H indicates *doing hills gently*. (Note: hills are bumps. If it's got "mount" in front of the name, like Mount Whitney, it's not a hill, it's a mountain!)

The reason for doing hills is for strength. The limiting factor for almost everyone in a half-marathon is that their legs start to tire and they slow right down. If you do hills, even gently, your legs get used to pushing and therefore don't tire as easily.

S means *speed training* (some of you won't have speed training on your program). But for those who do, S means that within the total workout time, an aspect of the training will be speed work, *not the entire workout.* If you refer to the key at the bottom right-hand corner of your program, it will provide the details on what to do.

C means *train either on the exact course* that the event will be on, or in conditions that are very similar to the course.

? beside a workout means that it's *optional*.

D/O means *take a day off*.

Note: If you are already running regularly, for longer times than are indicated at the beginning of the programs, you can just continue at that level for the first few weeks. When the training volumes start getting bigger and speed and hill workouts are added, start following the program. However, if you haven't had a break from training of at least two weeks in the last two years, then you really should start at the beginning—and, even better, take a week off before starting.

The training programs

Program 1: Walk

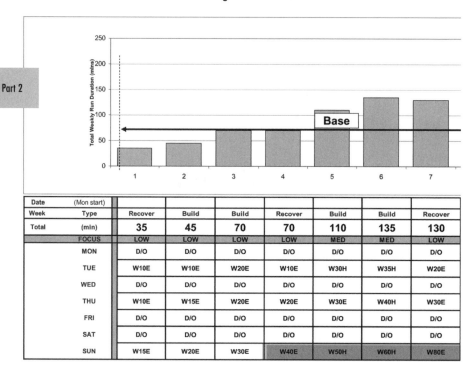

Date	(Mon start)						
Week	Type	Recover	Build	Build	Recover	Build	Build	Recover
Total	(min)	**35**	**45**	**70**	**70**	**110**	**135**	**130**
	FOCUS	LOW	LOW	LOW	LOW	MED	MED	LOW
	MON	D/O	D/O	D/O	D/O	D/O	D/O	D/O
	TUE	W10E	W10E	W20E	W10E	W30H	W35H	W20E
	WED	D/O	D/O	D/O	D/O	D/O	D/O	D/O
	THU	W10E	W15E	W20E	W20E	W30E	W40H	W30E
	FRI	D/O	D/O	D/O	D/O	D/O	D/O	D/O
	SAT	D/O	D/O	D/O	D/O	D/O	D/O	D/O
	SUN	W15E	W20E	W30E	W40E	W50H	W60H	W80E

Notes:

- Walks should be spaced Tu/Th/Su or similar to provide recovery time.
- It is OK to miss 10–20% of workouts. Try not to miss the longest walks.
- Don't train if you are not recovered—it will make you more tired or lead to injury.
- Start out slowly and comfortably to avoid injury. Most people get injured in the first four weeks by overdoing it.
- Take what you think is easy and slow down by at least another 20–30%, just for the first four weeks.
- Don't race people and overdo it—your challenge is to train smart enough not to get injured.
- Train on terrain similar to the course on the weekends—it will make it much easier on the day.

Part 2

Half-marathon training program

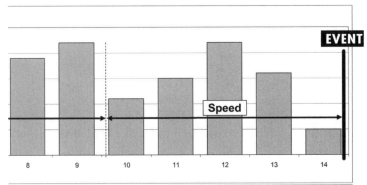

Build	Build	Recover	Build	Build	Recover	Recover
190	220	110	150	220	160	50
MED	MED	LOW	HIGH	HIGH	HIGH	HIGH
D/O	D/O	D/O	D/O	D/O	D/O	D/O
W40H	W40H	W30E	W20H	W40H	W30H	W30E
D/O	D/O	D/O	D/O	D/O	D/O	W10E
W50H	W60H	W20E	W30H	W60H	W40H	D/O
D/O	D/O	D/O	D/O	D/O	D/O	D/O
D/O	D/O	D/O	D/O	D/O	D/O	W10E
W100H	W120H	W60E	W100C	W120C	W90C	EVENT

Key:

E = EASY WALKING (easy conversation pace)
H = HILLS (easy walking on moderate hills)
C = TERRAIN LIKE THE COURSE
W = WALK
D/O = DAY OFF

All training volumes are in minutes.

Program 2: Walk/run

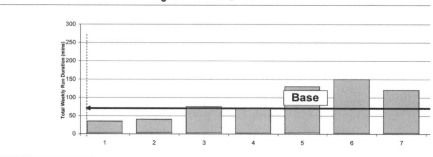

Date	(Mon start)						
Week	Type	Recover	Build	Build	Recover	Build	Build	Recover
Total	(min)	**35**	**40**	**75**	**70**	**130**	**150**	**120**
	FOCUS	LOW	LOW	LOW	LOW	MED	MED	LOW
MON		D/O	D/O	D/O	D/O	D/O	D/O	D/O
TUE		W10E	W10E	W10H	W10E	R30E	R30E	R20E
WED		D/O	D/O	D/O	D/O	D/O	D/O	D/O
THU		W10E	W10E	W15E	RW20E	RW20E	RW30H	RW30E
FRI		D/O	D/O	D/O	D/O	D/O	D/O	D/O
SAT		D/O	D/O	W10C	D/O	W20E	W30E	D/O
SUN		W15E	W20E	W30E	W40E	RW50H	RW60H	W70E

Notes:

- Walks/runs should be spaced Tu/Th/Sa/Su or similar to provide recovery time.
- It is OK to miss 10–20% of workouts. Try not to miss the longest runs.
- Don't train if you are not recovered—it will make you more tired or lead to injury.
- Start out slowly and comfortably to avoid injury. Most people get injured in the first four weeks by overdoing it.
- Take what you think is easy and slow down by at least another 20–30%, just for the first four weeks.
- Don't race people and overdo it—your challenge is to train smart enough not to get injured.
- Train on terrain similar to the course on the weekends—it will make it much easier on the day.

Half-marathon training program

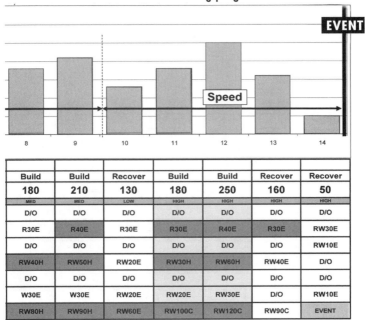

Part 2

Build	Build	Recover	Build	Build	Recover	Recover
180	**210**	**130**	**180**	**250**	**160**	**50**
MED	MED	LOW	HIGH	HIGH	HIGH	HIGH
D/O	D/O	D/O	D/O	D/O	D/O	D/O
R30E	R40E	R30E	R30E	R40E	R30E	RW30E
D/O	D/O	D/O	D/O	D/O	D/O	RW10E
RW40H	RW50H	RW20E	RW30H	RW60H	RW40E	D/O
D/O	D/O	D/O	D/O	D/O	D/O	D/O
W30E	W30E	RW20E	RW20E	RW30E	D/O	RW10E
RW80H	RW90H	RW60E	RW100C	RW120C	RW90C	EVENT

Key:

E =   EASY WALKING/RUNNING (easy conversation pace)
H =   HILLS (easy running/walking on moderate hills)
C =   TERRAIN LIKE THE COURSE
W =   WALK
R =   RUN
RW =   RUN AS MUCH AS YOU CAN COMFORTABLY AND WALK
        IN BETWEEN
D/O =   DAY OFF

All training volumes are in minutes.

Part 2

Program 3: Beginner run

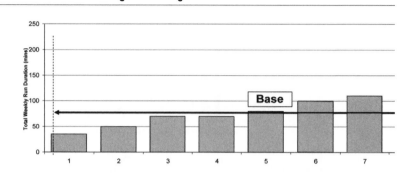

Date	(Mon start)							
Week	Type	Recover	Build	Build	Recover	Build	Build	Recover
Total	(min)	**35**	**50**	**70**	**70**	**80**	**100**	**110**
	FOCUS	LOW	LOW	LOW	LOW	MED	MED	LOW
MON		D/O	D/O	D/O	D/O	D/O	D/O	D/O
TUES		10E	15E	20H	20E	20H	30H	20E
WED		D/O	D/O	D/O	D/O	D/O	D/O	D/O
THURS		10E	15E	20E	20E	20H	20H	30E
FRI		D/O	D/O	D/O	D/O	D/O	D/O	D/O
SAT		D/O	D/O	D/O	D/O	D/O	D/O	D/O
SUN		15E	20E	30E	30C	40E	50E	60C

Notes:

- Runs should be spaced Tu/Th/Su or similar to provide recovery time.
- It is OK to miss 10–20% of workouts. Try not to miss the longest runs.
- Don't train if you are not recovered—it will make you more tired or lead to injury.
- If you do speed work, do it at the correct intensity. Doing speed work harder will not be beneficial, as it will be at the wrong intensity.
- Start out slowly and comfortably to avoid injury. Most people get injured in the first four weeks by overdoing it.
- Take what you think is easy and slow down by at least another 20–30%, just for the first four weeks.
- Don't race people and overdo it—your challenge is to train smart enough not to get injured.
- Train on terrain similar to the course on the weekends—it will make it much easier on the day.

Half-marathon training program

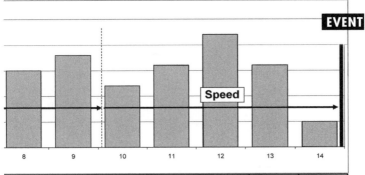

8	9	10	11	12	13	14
Build	Build	Recover	Build	Build	Recover	Recover
150	180	120	160	220	160	50
MED	MED	LOW	HIGH	HIGH	HIGH	HIGH
D/O	D/O	D/O	D/O	D/O	D/O	D/O
30H	40S	30E	30E	40S	30S	20E
D/O	D/O	D/O	D/O	D/O	D/O	20E
40H	50H	30E	30E	60H	40H	D/O
D/O	D/O	D/O	D/O	D/O	D/O	D/O
D/O	D/O	D/O	D/O	D/O	D/O	10E
80E	90E	60E	100E	120C	90C	EVENT

Key:

E =   EASY RUNNING (easy conversation pace)
H =   HILLS (easy running on moderate hills)
C =   TERRAIN LIKE THE COURSE
S =   SPEED (half-marathon pace, one to four x five minutes—no faster)
D/O = DAY OFF

NOTE: Half-marathon pace is the pace you think you will do the event at.

All training volumes are in minutes.

Part 2

Program 4: Improver run

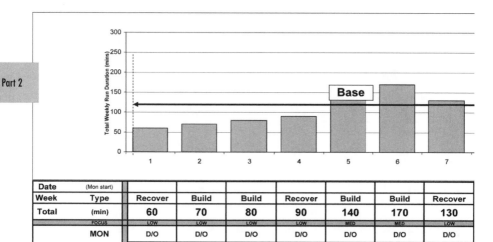

Date	(Mon start)							
Week	Type	Recover	Build	Build	Recover	Build	Build	Recover
Total	(min)	**60**	**70**	**80**	**90**	**140**	**170**	**130**
	FOCUS	LOW	LOW	LOW	LOW	MED	MED	LOW
MON		D/O	D/O	D/O	D/O	D/O	D/O	D/O
TUE		20E	20E	20H	20E	30H	30A	20E
WED		D/O	D/O	D/O	D/O	D/O	D/O	D/O
THU		20E	20E	20E	20E	30H	40H	30E
FRI		D/O	D/O	D/O	D/O	D/O	D/O	D/O
SAT		D/O	D/O	D/O	D/O	20E?	30E?	D/O
SUN		20E	30E	40E	50C	60H	70H	80C

Notes:

- Runs should be spaced Tu/Th/Sa/Su or similar to provide recovery time.
- It is OK to miss 10–20% of workouts. Try not to miss the longest runs.
- Don't train if you are not recovered—it will make you more tired or lead to injury.
- If you do speed work, do it at the correct intensity. Doing speed work harder will not be beneficial, as it will be at the wrong intensity.
- Start out slowly and comfortably to avoid injury. Most people get injured in the first four weeks by overdoing it.
- Take what you think is easy and slow down by at least another 20–30%, just for the first four weeks.
- Don't race people and overdo it—your challenge is to train smart enough not to get injured.
- Train on terrain similar to the course on the weekends—it will make it much easier on the day.

Half-marathon training program

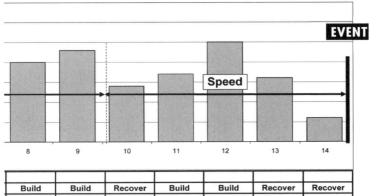

Build	Build	Recover	Build	Build	Recover	Recover
200	**230**	**140**	**170**	**250**	**160**	**60**
MED	MED	LOW	HIGH	HIGH	HIGH	HIGH
D/O	D/O	D/O	D/O	D/O	D/O	D/O
30A	40S	30S	30E	40S	30S	30E
D/O	D/O	D/O	D/O	D/O	D/O	20E
50H	60H	30E	30E	60H	40H	D/O
D/O	D/O	D/O	D/O	D/O	D/O	D/O
30E?	30E?	20E?	20C?	30C?	D/O	10E
90H	100H	60E	90E	120C	90C	EVENT

Key:

E =   EASY RUNNING (easy conversation pace)
H =   HILLS (easy running on moderate hills)
C =   TERRAIN LIKE THE COURSE
? =   OPTIONAL RUN (preferable that you do it)
A =   ACCELERATIONS (move up to half-marathon pace, hold until you start to puff, then back off and recover; one to six x 60 seconds)
S =   SPEED (half-marathon pace, one to four x five minutes—no faster)
D/O = DAY OFF

NOTE: Half-marathon pace is the pace you think you will do the event at.

All training volumes are in minutes.

Program 5: Competitive run

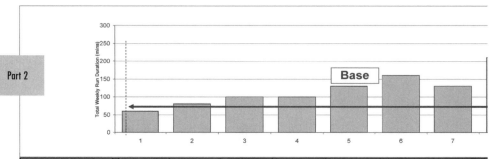

Date	(Mon start)							
Week	Type	Recover	Build	Build	Recover	Build	Build	Recover
Total	(min)	**60**	**80**	**100**	**100**	**130**	**160**	**130**
	FOCUS	LOW	LOW	LOW	LOW	MED	MED	LOW
	MON	D/O	D/O	D/O	D/O	D/O	D/O	D/O
	TUE	20E	20E	30H + He	20E	30H + He	30H + He	20H
	WED	D/O	D/O	D/O	D/O	D/O	D/O	D/O
	THU	20E	30E	30E	30E	20H + He	30H + He	30E
	FRI	D/O	D/O	D/O	D/O	D/O	D/O	D/O
	SAT	D/O	D/O	D/O	D/O	20C?	30C?	D/O
	SUN	20E	30E	40H	50C	60H	70H	80TT

Notes:

- Runs should be spaced Tu/Th/Sa/Su or similar to provide recovery time.
- It is OK to miss 10–20% of workouts. Try not to miss the longest runs.
- Don't train if you are not recovered—it will make you more tired or lead to injury.
- If you do speed work, do it at the correct intensity. Doing speed work harder will not be beneficial, as it will be at the wrong intensity.
- Start out slowly and comfortably to avoid injury. Most people get injured in the first four weeks by overdoing it.
- Take what you think is easy and slow down by at least another 20–30%, just for the first four weeks.
- Don't race people and overdo it—your challenge is to train smart enough not to get injured.
- Train on terrain similar to the course on the weekends—it will make it much easier on the day.

Half-marathon training program

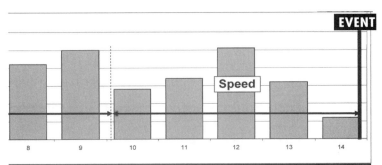

Part 2

Build	Build	Recover	Build	Build	Recover	Recover
210	**250**	**140**	**170**	**255**	**160**	**60**
MED	MED	LOW	HIGH	HIGH	HIGH	HIGH
D/O	D/O	D/O	D/O	D/O	D/O	D/O
40H + He	40H + He	30H	30S**	45S**	30S**	30E
D/O	D/O	D/O	D/O	D/O	D/O	20E
40H + He	60H + He	30E	30E	60H + He	40H + He	D/O
D/O	D/O	D/O	D/O	D/O	D/O	D/O
30C?	30C?	20E	20S*	30S*	D/O	10E
100H	120H	60TT	90H	120C	90C	EVENT

Key:

E = EASY RUNNING (easy conversation pace)

H = HILLS (easy running on moderate hills)

C = TERRAIN LIKE THE COURSE

He = HILL EFFORTS (run up a gradual incline—2%—at half-marathon pace, one to six x 200 m)

TT = 6 km TIME TRIAL (at half-marathon pace—no faster!)

S* = SPEED (half-marathon pace, one to four x five minutes)

S** = SPEED (slightly faster than half-marathon pace— one to four x 30 seconds. Only *slightly* faster!)

? = OPTIONAL RUN (preferable that you do it)

D/O = DAY OFF

NOTE: Half-marathon pace is the pace you think you will do the event at.

All training volumes are in minutes.

Program 6: Race

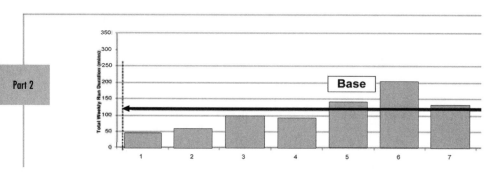

Date	(Mon start)							
Week	Type	Recover	Build	Build	Recover	Build	Build	Recover
Total	(min)	**70**	**80**	**120**	**110**	**140**	**200**	**130**
	FOCUS	LOW	LOW	LOW	LOW	MED	MED	LOW
MON		D/O	D/O	D/O	D/O	D/O	D/O	D/O
TUES		20H	20H	20H + He	30E	30H + He	30H + He	20H
WED		D/O	D/O	D/O	D/O	20E	20E	D/O
THURS		20E	30E	30H	30E	30H + He	40H + He	30E
FRI		D/O	D/O	D/O	D/O	D/O	D/O	D/O
SAT		D/O	D/O	30C	D/O	20C	30C	20E
SUN		30E	30E	40H	50E	60H	80H	60TT

Notes:

- Runs should be spaced Tu/Th/Sa/Su or similar to provide recovery time.
- It is OK to miss 10–20% of workouts. Try not to miss the longest runs.
- Don't train if you are not recovered—it will make you more tired or lead to injury.
- If you do speed work, do it at the correct intensity. Doing speed work harder will not be beneficial, as it will be at the wrong intensity.
- Start out slowly and comfortably to avoid injury. Most people get injured in the first four weeks by overdoing it.
- Take what you think is easy and slow down by at least another 20–30%, just for the first four weeks.
- Don't race people and overdo it—your challenge is to train smart enough not to get injured.
- Train on terrain similar to the course on the weekends—it will make it much easier on the day.

Half-marathon training program

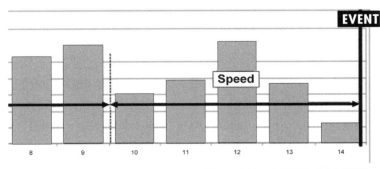

Build	Build	Recover	Build	Build	Recover	Recover
260	**300**	**150**	**190**	**310**	**180**	**60**
MED	MED	LOW	HIGH	HIGH	HIGH	HIGH
D/O	D/O	D/O	D/O	D/O	D/O	D/O
40S*	50S*	30H	30E	50S*	30S*	30E
30E	30E	D/O	20E	30E	D/O	20E
60H + He	70H + He	30E	30H + He	80H + He	40H	D/O
D/O	D/O	D/O	D/O	D/O	D/O	D/O
30C	30S**	30E	20S**	30S**	20S**	10E
100H	120H	60TT	90H	120C	90C	EVENT

Key:

E = EASY RUNNING (easy conversation pace)
H = HILLS (easy running on moderate hills)
C = TERRAIN LIKE THE COURSE
He = HILL EFFORTS (run up a gradual incline—2%—at half-marathon pace, one to six x 200 m)
TT = 8 km TIME TRIAL (at half-marathon pace—no faster!)
S* = SPEED (half-marathon pace, one to four x five minutes)
S** = SPEED (slightly faster than half-marathon pace— one to four x 30 seconds. Only *slightly* faster!)
? = OPTIONAL RUN (preferable that you do it)
D/O = DAY OFF

NOTE: Half-marathon pace is the pace you think you will do the event at.

All training volumes are in minutes.

CHAPTER 9

Using your training program effectively: What's key and what's not

OK, so now you have a program and an understanding of how to use it. The next step is to understand that there are two parts to the training equation.

You have to have a good plan (your training program) but you also have to be able to use the plan well. You can't have a program and think, "Great, I'm set now." You need to control your training.

Here's how you do it. While the whole program is important, all parts are not created equal. You need to understand two big issues:

1. how to last the distance; and

2. some workouts are more important than others.

LASTING THE DISTANCE

When the majority of people are given a new training program, how much energy do you think they immediately put into it? They are super enthusiastic, the training is new and exciting so . . .

You guessed it: they give it *tons*!

The question then is, by the time they get to the end of the training program, how much energy do they have left for the event they have been training for?

As you might guess, *not much*!

It's extremely easy to get overexcited at the start of your training program. But if you start your program too hard or with too much enthusiasm you may find your energy running out before you get to the event.

So, break your program into thirds. You want to start *lazy*, go to *diligent*, and end up *focused*. Yes, you read that correctly. Lazy, diligent, focused.

As discussed in Chapter 5, your body adapts to each new, slightly harder training bout whether it's due to an increase in the duration, the amount of hill work or the speed. So as you go through the training, your body is adapting to higher and higher requirements.

The last few weeks, when the requirements are at their maximum, just before your training tapers down, is where you finally get the training adaptation that helps you to do well in the event. All the training prior to this time just puts you in condition to deal with the last weeks of training. Saving your energy for those important last few weeks allows you to get the best results. You don't want to be winding down and pooped just when it really matters.

An exercise example will illustrate this idea further. If you lift a weight ten to 12 times (until your muscles won't lift any more), which of the ten to 12 repetitions actually generate the strength? Well, generally it's the last couple. Those are the key repetitions. The first eight to ten reps just put you in a position to get a result from the last couple.

The same applies to your training program. The weeks that really count are the last two building weeks in the entire program. Everything prior to that is just preparation for those key weeks!

You will not be in a condition to get the most out of those key weeks if, like most people, you start off psychotic, move to exhausted, and end up a small lump of charcoal just at the time when you're doing your key training weeks. In other words, just when you should be getting all those performance gains at the end of the training program, you will be too tired to absorb the training and so your performance will either plateau or get worse.

Part 2

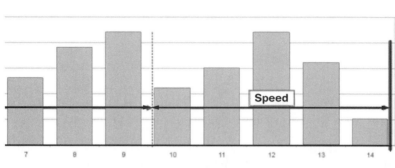

Recover	Build	Build	Recover	Build	Build	Recover	Recover
130	**190**	**220**	**110**	**150**	**220**	**160**	**50**
LOW	MED	MED	LOW	HIGH	HIGH	HIGH	HIGH
D/O	D/O	D/O	D/O	D/O	D/O	D/O	D/O
W20E	W40H	W40H	W30E	W20H	W40H	W30H	W30E
D/O	D/O	D/O	D/O	D/O	D/O	D/O	W10E
W30E	W50H	W60H	W20E	W30H	W60H	W40H	D/O
D/O	D/O	D/O	D/O	D/O	D/O	D/O	D/O
D/O	D/O	D/O	D/O	D/O	D/O	D/O	W10E
W80E	W100H	W120H	W60E	W100C	W120C	W90C	EVENT

These final key weeks are highlighted above for you, in grey. This is what we call *focus control*.

KEY IS THE KEY

The next thing to talk about is the 80/20 rule. The 80/20 rule states that 80% of your result comes from 20% of your activities. If you apply that rule to business, it means 80% of your revenue comes from 20% of your clients. Or 80% of orders in a restaurant come from 20% of the items on the menu.

When it comes to training, 80% of your performance improvement comes from 20% of your training. The key is to understand *which 20% of training is going to give you that 80% return*. These vital few workouts control most of your fitness improvement.

This means that there are workouts that you can miss and there are workouts that you don't want to miss. The trick is to try to move from key workout to key workout. Get the training done in between but try to keep yourself ready for the next key workout, because that is where most of your improvements are coming from.

The most important workouts are usually your longest and second-longest runs or walks for the week. They are highlighted in grey on the training programs (see below). You want to try to do each of these well even if you have to forgo a few other smaller workouts to achieve this.

So let's say you've just done your long run for the week: your key workout. You should immediately start to think about your next key workout, your second-longest run for the week. It will be a few days away so you should do the training that is scheduled for the days in between only if you are sure that you can still be ready to do a good job in the next key workout.

Once again you have your priorities straight in terms of return on effort—keep training smart!

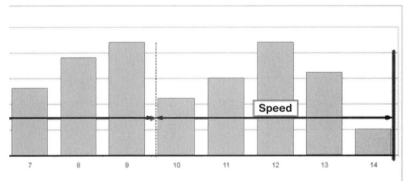

Recover	Build	Build	Recover	Build	Build	Recover	Recover
130	**190**	**220**	**110**	**150**	**220**	**160**	**50**
LOW	MED	MED	LOW	HIGH	HIGH	HIGH	HIGH
D/O	D/O	D/O	D/O	D/O	D/O	D/O	D/O
W20E	W40H	W40H	W30E	W20H	W40H	W30H	W30E
D/O	D/O	D/O	D/O	D/O	D/O	D/O	W10E
W30E	W50H	W60H	W20E	W30H	W60H	W40H	D/O
D/O	D/O	D/O	D/O	D/O	D/O	D/O	D/O
D/O	D/O	D/O	D/O	D/O	D/O	D/O	W10E
W80E	W100H	W120H	W60E	W100C	W120C	W90C	EVENT

Working through your program week by week

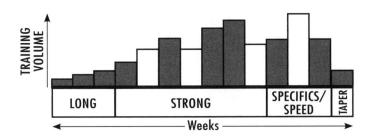

Read each chapter at the relevant time as you work through your program. Each chapter will discuss issues pertinent to what you are doing and experiencing at that time, and should answer most of your questions.

CHAPTER 10

Before you start:

Controlling the mental game

As well as the training, there is also "the game." How you play the game is very important. And the game does not start when the gun goes off on race day. No, no, no . . . the game starts as soon as you decide to do the event.

How is the game played?

Well, imagine the half-marathon is a person, and that person is trying to beat you . . . trying to stop you from starting the event, trying to stop you finishing, trying to sabotage the enjoyment you will experience as you take on this challenge. This is what you are up against!

What negative tactics will the event use to try to beat you?

Negative tactic number 1: misinformation

Did you know that everybody's a training expert? You will find this out as soon as you start training. All sorts of people will give you all sorts of information on how to train, how often to train, and how fast to train. Unfortunately, much of this information will confuse or mislead you.

Others will ask you questions like: "How many miles are you running/ walking each week?" "How long is your longest run/walk?" or "How much speed work are you doing?" Whatever answer you give will be greeted with a raised eyebrow, a story about how they did it, or a prediction about the trouble that lies ahead.

Don't get me wrong: these people mostly have good intentions. But the end result, if you don't have control, is a serious dose of "I'm not sure what to do."

Negative tactic number 2: self-doubt

The event, with a little help from its friends, will plant seeds of doubt at every opportunity. It will even water them if you give it a chance!

For example, you will know the game is winning if you are asking yourself questions like: "Have I done enough training?" "Can I do this?" or "Am I getting more fit?"

Negative tactic number 3: more self-doubt

Have you done every workout on the program, no matter what? Are you dragging one leg back into the house? Is your wife/husband/significant other saying: "Are you sure you're all right?" and you're saying, "I'm fine," even though you're bleeding from the ears?

Are you running despite your Achilles tendon feeling like it has a hot poker stuck in it? Are you running at 10:30 at night to get your workouts in? Are you turning every workout into a time trial? Has your dog seen so little of you recently that it thinks you are an intruder?

If you answer yes to any of these, you have lost control and the event is winning!

Negative tactic number 4: pressure (first-timers only)

People—bad people—will ask you: "What time are you going to do?"
Now, it's likely if you are reading this book that you have never run or
walked a half-marathon before. You may not have even seen the course
before. Yet what do you do when people ask you what time you are going
to do?

Right, you give them a time.

Big, bad mistake! All this does is put pressure on you (and the event loves
you to do this).

When it comes to your time, relax, especially if it's your first half-marathon.
On the day, all you have to do is turn up, stick to the plan on the day, and
enjoy the moment. Your time will take care of itself.

If you do this, when you cross the finish line, not only will you have met the
challenge of completing a half-marathon, you will have controlled the event.

You have a choice: either you control the event, or the event controls you.
Stay in control!

Don't sweat the misses

Another common mistake people make when they get a new training
program is thinking that it is critical that they do every workout. Some even
believe that if they miss one workout the whole program will be blown
apart!

Here's the good news: *we expect you to miss 10 to 20% of the training
program*. Therefore, if life gets in the way of training, don't sweat it. The
program will still do its job (remember the "I've got a life outside running"
example in Chapter 6).

However, if you are missing more than 20% of the workouts on your
program, then you need to look again at whether training for this event is
feasible, or whether you need to be a little more disciplined. If you're
missing less than 10% you also need to stop and think, because either the
program's perfect, your life's perfect, or most likely you need to deal with
the word "obsession"!

DOING THE NUMBERS VS. HOW YOU FEEL

There's a big difference between "doing the numbers" on the program and doing the training. Doing the numbers means going out and doing what is written on the program, regardless of how you feel. Doing the training means going out only when you feel good enough to absorb the training and get a performance gain. In other words, you ask yourself: when is it worth training and when is it a waste of time?

Listen to your body and trust what it's telling you. If you feel tired and you're not looking forward to training, head out the door and see if that feeling passes. If you're still looking for your enthusiasm after about five or ten minutes, then it's probably better to go home and put your feet up. Tomorrow is another day!

The simplest question to ask yourself is: Am I the same or better in this workout than I was in the "like" workout last week?

If the answer is I'm the same, that's OK—you can't improve every time.

If the answer is I'm better, great—pat yourself on the back.

If the answer is I'll be worse, it means that you are too tired to do a good job today. Go home and recover!

So, you're about to start on the program. You know how to handle it, so start gently as we begin to work through the 14 weeks. Resist the temptation to add more duration to your workouts—this will come with time.

When you run or walk you lose fluid through sweat and breathing. You need to replace this during longer bouts of exercise or in hot conditions. I would drink two to three mouthfuls of sports fluid replacement drink approximately every 15 minutes during exercise as a rule of thumb—more if it's a hot day and less if it's cooler. Starting a workout a little dehydrated will mean an impaired ability to perform at your usual levels, which decreases the "fitness returns" you get out of the workout.

It will also make the workout more uncomfortable because your physical state is worse. It could even be harmful to your health if you get too dehydrated. The fluid in your bloodstream, which is replenished by drinking, is like the oil in your car—if the level gets too low, the engine seizes! Drink a little often to ensure that your training is effective.

My last suggestion before you start—and probably the most important advice I can give to reduce your chances of injury—is to do as much of your early training off-road as you can, especially on grass and trails that have a firm footing. Running or walking on concrete has several disadvantages in early training. The impact on your legs is greater due to the harder surface, and the uniformity of the terrain causes your feet, knees and hips to "track" identically with each step over and over again, which overloads specific parts of your leg muscles. It might be that the outside of your knee begins to give you trouble or the muscle behind your hip bone starts to ache. Running or walking on slightly rolling grass or trails causes your legs to "track" slightly differently with each step. With slightly varied differences in the running surface under your feet, the load is spread more evenly around your leg muscles. This reduces wear and load in specific areas, which reduces injury and keeps your legs fresher. Run or walk off-road, particularly on your longer workouts. As you get closer to a road-running event, start to move your longer runs onto the road, with the second-longest run being phased onto the road about 8 weeks before the event and your longest run joining this with 6 or 5 weeks to go. This is the best anti-injury advice.

CHAPTER 11

WEEK ONE

Basic proper technique

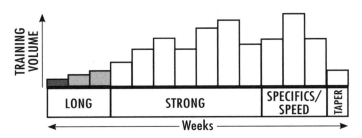

SHOWING YOUR BODY HOW TO PERFORM THE ACTIONS

If you can run or walk efficiently, all you need to be able to do is perform this action correctly again and again and again for the distance of the event. This is endurance or "going long." Endurance is your ability to maintain good technique for the duration of the event. Before you build up your endurance, you need to start with technique, as being unable to run or walk properly makes training very difficult!

Although you may have practiced walking or running all your life, it might surprise you to know that with an understanding of a few basic pointers you can get much better, literally overnight.

Why bother?

Well, having good technique means a lower chance of injury. It also means you tire more slowly in the event—i.e. you'll feel stronger for longer, and therefore it helps you perform better and have a fun, successful day. Not bad for a few quick pointers!

I often see people out for a run or a walk and see them struggling through their workout. I want to rush over and tell them I know how to make things easier, but I don't—nobody likes a wise guy. In this case, though, it's my book, and I'm assuming you're interested, so here are some tips.

Part 3
Week 1

Performing the actions correctly

The first thing you need to show your body are the actions required in the event, in this case running or walking. If it thinks it's kayaking or horseback riding, you've made a serious mistake!

You don't have to show your body anything else, you just go out there and you run, or you walk. You're doing very small volumes and you're starting out nice and gently. Your body receives the first part of the picture.

So what can you do to improve your technique? How can you make yourself better, by making a few small changes that will make your training easier?

BALANCE

The most important thing to do is learn to balance the vertical weight of your body on your skeleton. A lot of runners or walkers exercise with poor technique, either all the time or when they get tired. They will tend to either "sit in the bucket" or they lean forward. This means that extra body weight is carried by their muscles rather than their bones, increasing predisposition to injury, reducing their speed and making them tire and slow down significantly towards the end of the event.

Imagine balancing a broom handle vertically in the palm of your open hand, with the brush pointing up to the sky. If you run or walk forward, the broom has to lean forward slightly to remain balanced.

Imagine that your spine is the broom handle and try and balance it on your pelvis. If you can sense this you can have perfect running or walking balance.

Think of the "broom handle" technique, stand tall when you run or walk and look at your reflection in windows that you pass to check that your shoulders are over your hips. Your shoulders should be either directly over your hips or a half to three-quarters of an inch in front of your hips depending on the speed you are running or walking at (the faster you are running or walking, the further forwards your shoulders will be).

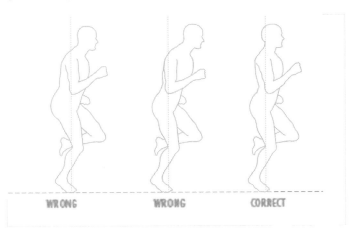

WRONG   WRONG   CORRECT

The second trick is to keep your chin up, which also helps to keep your body upright. If you drop your head you will tend to lean forward and start to run on your toes.

Be particularly vigilant about balance late in a workout. Bad technique often creeps in as you start to tire. It's a good idea to pull your cap down so that the brim obscures your vision slightly. This means that if you don't keep your chin up you won't be able to see where you are going. Lamp-posts don't tend to get out of the way!

For this week, work on running or walking gently and getting your body accustomed to exercise. Next week we will start thinking about technique in your training.

CHAPTER 12

WEEK TWO

Advanced technique

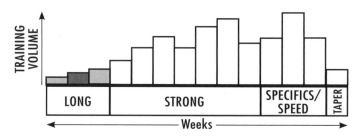

Now that we have been training for a couple of weeks, it's time to refine technique.

FLUIDITY—ELIMINATING INTERFERENCE TO SPEED

Fluidity is about eliminating any interference to the power and effort you put out. If you run incorrectly you can cause a braking effect on every stride.

Fluidity technique tip number 1

Your foot should contact the ground directly underneath your body. If your foot lands ahead of your body there is a braking effect, which will slow you down and cause your legs to fatigue faster.

You also cannot effectively apply force until your pelvis is directly over your feet. So if your foot contacts the ground ahead of your body there is a split second where you lose momentum.

In a half-marathon most people will take one stride per yard or approximately 21,000 strides over the entire event. If your technique means you are interrupting momentum and braking on every stride, that is a lot of wasted energy!

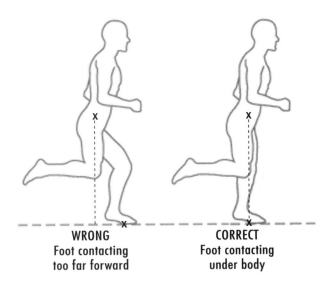

<table>
<tr><td align="center">**WRONG**
Foot contacting
too far forward</td><td align="center">**CORRECT**
Foot contacting
under body</td></tr>
</table>

Part 3
Week 2

Fluidity technique tip number 2

Your foot should contact the ground at the same speed as your body is moving over the ground. If your foot contacts the ground more slowly—say at 10 min/mile when you are running at 8 min/mile—there is a braking effect.

Ideally, the combination of the first two fluidity tips makes your footfall virtually silent. Often you will notice that as you get progressively more fatigued in a long workout, your footfall becomes louder.

Also, try not to bounce up and down. This vertical effort is wasted; you want to direct as much of your effort into horizontal speed. Once again, look at how you run in windows that you pass and try to remove the bounce.

Fluidity technique tip number 3

You also need to think about your arm swing. Your arms should move forward and back in line with where you are going, opposite arm to leg. Your arms should gently piston forward and back, not across your body. Your elbows should be bent at an 80 to 90 degree angle and your shoulders and face should be relaxed. Running or walking with your hands open will help relax your arms and shoulders.

Stable platform

Finally, good core stability will help you to run or walk faster. Having strong abdominal muscles will tend to hold your pelvis more firmly, allowing all your effort to be put onto the road rather than being partially lost as your pelvis "gives" by rocking or dropping. Talk to a personal trainer or someone at the gym about strengthening your core stability.

Try thinking about one of these technique tips each time you exercise, and alternate them through your workouts.

CHAPTER 13

WEEK THREE

Building strength

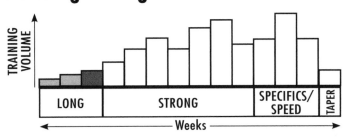

As you might have guessed, the limiting factor in a half-marathon is not your lungs, it's your legs. There is very little chance that you will run out of breath but your legs may turn to stone.

People talk about half-marathons as being endurance events, but they're not: they're *strength endurance* events. Think about that for a moment. This difference is important because it will dictate what we show your body in training. We will focus on training the power in your legs while doing your workouts and we focus on looking after your legs during the event.

To improve strength endurance in your legs, we provide a lot of resistance work in your training program to get your legs conditioned to "pushing" for long periods of time. *This is probably the most important aspect of your training*—do not underestimate it.

So how do we do this? In the second third of your training program, we will give you hills to do in your workouts. You will run or walk hills, and when you are not doing hills you do hills, and when you are not doing hills or hills we will work on doing—you guessed it—hills.

Now you might be thinking, "Oh, I don't want to (or can't!) do hills." But don't forget, you won't do lots of hills until you are a long way into the program. By the time you get to this part of the program you'll have a tattoo saying "I love hills."

Start to incorporate hill work into your workouts, where stated. Run or walk hills gently and remember to reduce your stride length and use baby steps when going up hills.

As you progress through the next few weeks, try to gradually increase the amount of hills you gently do in each hill workout.

**Part 3
Week 3**

CHAPTER 14

WEEK FOUR

Knowing the course

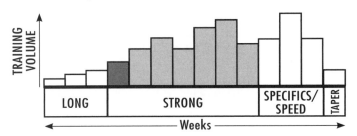

By week four you should be coming out of the most difficult phase of the program. The first four weeks are where you are most likely to become injured. If there are still a few problems please refer to the "troubleshooting" reference section at the end of this book.

Fluids

As the training mileage increases it becomes more important to hydrate (which is a way of saying you need to have a drink due to the length of time you are exercising). At this point it is worth finding out (if you can) what the race fluid used in the event is. For most big events this will be available on the website long before the big day. See if you can purchase and use the product during your training so as to adapt your stomach to it.

The reason this is important is that on the big day you will probably be a little nervous, which can upset your stomach.

As you begin to get tired during the event, the fatigue can also make your stomach sensitive. If it's a hot day, the slight increase in body temperature can also lead to a more sensitive stomach.

The last thing that you want to do on the day is put a drink in your stomach that you have never experienced before or adapted to. Potentially this can lead to mild nausea all the way to causing you to empty your stomach contents onto the road, which is not pleasant or pretty, and likely means there will be no hugs and kisses at the finish line, if you know what I mean.

Another useful idea as the distances in your training become longer is to get some sort of "hydration pack" or belt to carry fluid with you when you exercise. You will find this at your local running or sporting goods store.

Never mess with someone you know very little about!

There is an old cliché that says:

"Never mess with someone you don't know."

Part 3
Week 4

You don't know what they know or what they can do so there is a chance you will end up in trouble.

The same thinking can also be applied to an event. If you can, start to learn as much as you can about the event.

Initially you might

- ↓ go to the website
- ↓ start asking people who have done the event before
- ↓ ask experienced runners
- ↓ ask coaches

You want to get a feel for what you will be messing with on the "big day."

The better you understand what you are in for, the more accurately you can "mimic" what you will encounter during the event!

On the website, look at the course map and hill profile. Try to get an understanding of what the event might be like. This will tell you whether it is hilly or flat and whether there are any major obstacles that might need a bit of thinking about. If the event is in a hot climate (more than 8–10° F hotter than where you normally train) it might be worth putting on extra clothes in the final three weeks of training to simulate the heat. You want to know what the likelihood of a cold or windy day is so you can get the right clothing to deal with this.

Training on the course:

+ If you possibly can, it is worth visiting the course and training on it at least once before the big day.
+ If you live close by, regularly do your long runs on the course.
+ If you're traveling from a greater distance away, try to run on the course five and three weeks out from the event day on your long runs.
+ If you can only run on it once, go three weeks before the event.
+ If you cannot run on the course at all, try to arrive two to three days early and do some of your final short runs on the course and drive it to get a sense of what it will be like.

Knowing the course has some hidden performance benefits to make your life easier.

If I said I want you to do a 6 mile time trial on a course you know and a 6 mile time trial on a course you don't know, which one would you go faster on? The answer is obvious: you will go faster on the course you know. This means the better you know the course, the better and more enjoyable your event day.

Part 3
Week 4

The key thing is to understand where all the landmarks are as you go through the event. The better you know the landmarks, the more you will have a sense of progress, and the more likely you are to feel positive and be able to pace yourself correctly. The key areas are the featureless areas of the course, particularly in the third quarter of the event. This is where most people start to feel a little despondent and potentially feel as if they are running "up a hill and don't know where the top is."

By event morning you should be able to tell the person next to you what the weather forecast for the event is, have the right clothing for this and know what all the big "crunch points" are on the course. The crunch points are the areas on the course that you have to pay particular attention to. These might be:

+ being careful about not starting too fast
+ paying particular attention to keeping your stride rate even on a big hill

⬇ not over striding on a downhill
⬇ reminding yourself to really concentrate on your running form as you begin to get tired

If you sat down with someone the day before and they said,

"Hi [insert your name], can you tell me a little bit about the event tomorrow?"

You would say,

"Sure, let's go and have lunch."

They would say,

"Why do we need to go and have lunch?"

You would say,

**Part 3
Week 4**

"Because it's going to take me that long to explain that all to you."

The full explanation of the course might take 30 minutes!

In other words, if someone asks you to tell them about the course, your answer is:

"Which 500 yards are talking about?"

You know the course that well. Training is about specifically preparing for your goal. The only way you do this is to train specifically for *your goal* half-marathon which is very different for training for *any* half-marathon. Be really specific. Think of yourself as a military general about to go into battle, as if your life depended on it. Think it through, start to work out how to best handle the event. It's not just the "brawn" that you use, it's the "brains." And the only way to do that is to understand the nature of what you're about to do. Start to compile a knowledge base over these next ten weeks on how to do a half-marathon and also how you would do a half-marathon on that particular course. Also think about what will happen the night before and what will end up happening on the morning leading up to the event. You will end up producing a simple "event plan" in your head so that the whole event is pre-choreographed before you even start.

CHAPTER 15

WEEK FIVE

Listening to your body

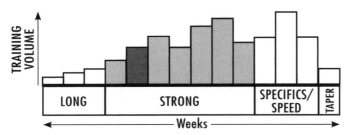

As you move into week five of the program the novelty of the training is wearing off and you are now in a situation where the training volume is starting to increase to more significant levels. It is time that we discuss dealing with enemy numero uno, fatigue!

Your ability to control fatigue decides how much of the training program you can do, whether you get injured, how well you do the training, whether you can last the distance and finish your program, and may even have an impact on whether you get sick!

Here's how. As you train, your body does its best to help. It is constantly telling you what it wants.

It is easy for most runners to ignore this and stay focused on "checking off" the next workout, completely disregarding their body's input.

Runners talk about "listening to their body" but most don't!

Your body is so clever in communicating its physical status to you, in that not only will it tell you to back off, it will even tell you specifically what to back off. Here's how:

→ If you are training too hard, the day after a workout, your body will have sore legs. It will say "Hey, back off, I'm tired and by the way, you are overtraining your muscles!"

> You are overtraining your muscular system.

→ If you do too much, say a really long run (twice the duration that is in your program for that workout), your body will have an elevated resting heart rate the next morning and you will "puff" walking up a flight of stairs. Your body will say "Back off, I'm tired and you went too far."

> You are overtraining the cardiovascular system.

→ If you've been going for too long, training month after month after month, you will lose enthusiasm. Once again your body says "Stop! I'm pooped, you've been training for too many months in a row, let's have a rest."

> You're overtraining the nervous system.

Let's say you don't listen to your body's signals.

→ You do too many hills and your body responds by giving you sore legs. But you keep going, training hills day after day. What happens next?

> You get injured!

→ What if you do huge training workouts day after day even though your body is giving you the signals to back off, like an elevated resting heart rate. What happens next?

> You get sick.

I know some people reading this will be saying "that's garbage," but why is it that you can put 200 people in a room, one has a cold and only 20 people catch the cold? Are those 20 the ones who spent the most time with the person with the cold, or are they the ones with the run down immune systems due to fatigue and are more susceptible to catching it?

↓ If you go month after month and your performance starts to drop and you do what "most people" do—you train harder—you will end with chronic fatigue syndrome or a mystery virus which no one can diagnose, which lasts for months, which just means that you are a smoldering wreck.

So when you train, your body gives you signals through fatigue. If you keep training regardless and don't listen, your body throws in the towel by becoming ill or injured. Remember, not listening during any conversation generally gets you into trouble!

Training is usually about improving. If you are not going to get better in today's workout, don't go out, wait until you can go out and get better.

So to summarize, performance is made up of non-verbal communication with your body. You show your body, through your actions, what you want it to prepare to do and it will tell you when to back off.

Make sure you are fresh enough to train well. This is covered by the question raised in Week 1:

"Am the same or better in this workout than I was in the 'like' workout last week?"

Training is about improving: if you are not the same or better then you haven't recovered and today's workout is not worth doing!

What to do: (monitoring fatigue)

Symptoms	Response
Heavy or sore legs	Cut down on the amount of hill work/hill efforts you are doing or do it more gently until you recover.
Elevated heart rate (puffing more)	Too much training, cut back on the number of workouts until you recover

Plateau in improvement Loss of enthusiasm	You have been training too many months in a row. Have a two week break if you can. There may be too much going on in other aspects of your life—either rearrange some things so life is a little less demanding or back off and do some light training until the busy period is over.

Remember a lot of the success in the event you are training for is based on how well you control your training, which is about training at the correct efforts so you don't end up being too tired to train, and knowing when to back off, or not train. This is your challenge, listen!

Monitoring Fatigue

Refer back to Chapter 2 and make sure you know your resting heart rate. Take your resting heart rate regularly during your training program, and if it goes up by more than 10%, this is a sign that you are cardio vascularly fatigued. Back off on the training and allow your body to recover for a few days until your resting heart rate returns to normal.

CHAPTER 16

WEEK SIX

Leg speed and rhythm

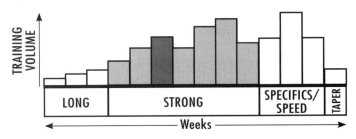

Now that your technique has improved, your training duration has come up and your strength is being worked on, let's discuss the next key area. There is another skill we now want to begin to work on which also has quite an impact on the final result.

LEG SPEED

Your leg speed is the speed at which you turn your legs over. This is often known as *stride rate*. For faster runners and shorter-distance events this should be up around 180 strides per minute, and for longer events this should drop to 170 strides per minute in most cases. For walkers it is more like 84 to 124 strides per minute, depending on age, size and conditioning. The key is to pick a stride rate that you can consistently maintain.

In addition to stride rate you have *stride length*, which is the distance you travel per stride. Your speed is a function of your stride length multiplied by your stride rate (e.g. stride length 1 yard x stride rate 180 strides per minute = 180 yards/min speed).

Most inexperienced runners tend to run with too low a stride rate. This means that they are taking too long a stride for their ability, which causes their legs to tire prematurely and is unpleasant and painful.

Combining a low stride rate with a longer stride than you can maintain is like bounding up flights of stairs in the Empire State Building three steps at a time. You'll look great for three or four flights and then your legs will start to "blow up."

Stride length is predominantly muscular: basically, the longer your stride length the more your muscles have to work. The higher your stride rate the more you require "puff." There is an unlimited supply of oxygen on all parts of the course, whereas you only have a limited amount of energy stored in your muscles. Once it runs very low, you are in trouble. This is what "hitting the wall" in a marathon is all about.

As most people become tired, their stride rate will often slow. This is noticeable at first on the hills and then later on the flat terrain. The key is, as you get tired, *reduce stride length but keep stride rate up at all costs*.

**Part 3
Week 6**

In a half-marathon, I can tell when a runner is going to start walking. If I listen to their footfall on the flat terrain I can hear the speed at which their stride rate is turning over. If they get to a hill and the rate of their footfall drops significantly, I know they'll be forced to walk soon.

Try to keep your stride rate consistent and take "baby steps" up the hills. Hills are where you need to focus on maintaining stride rate—particularly important towards the end of an event.

Rhythm

Try to keep the rhythm of your stride rate the same throughout the event. Once you break rhythm it is hard to get back, and the more fatigued you are the harder it is to get back! The event is going to try to break your rhythm if it can.

On the average half-marathon course, there will be somewhere between ten and 50 situations where you can have your rhythm broken. These are on hills, around corners or cones, through aid stations and when someone cuts in front of you.

During your training, try to get your stride rate up to approximately the stated frequencies, with a particular emphasis on maintaining this on hills. After an adaptation period you will find that you run or walk better, more comfortably and faster over longer distances.

Also practice maintaining your stride rate when you are out training so that you are ready for this in the event. This is surprisingly important to how well you do the event and how you feel while doing it.

CHAPTER 17

WEEK SEVEN

Technique adjustments

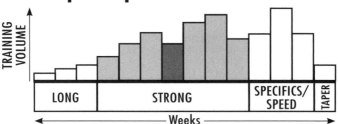

Here are a few more things to think about when it comes to technique. These are generalized so try them out and see if each area works for you. If it feels better, retain the technique and keep working on it. If it doesn't feel right, don't worry. Not everyone runs exactly the same, and you need to do what feels right.

Shoulders

Your shoulders should be low and relaxed. Often as a runner tires their shoulders creep up. This can slightly affect your ability to take in the oxygen that is so important, as your diaphragm tightens up. It can also lead to headaches and clenching your fists too tight.

> Action: Later in a run or event, monitor the tension in your shoulders and try and keep them relaxed. If you feel them tightening, drop your arms to your sides and shake the tension out.

Torso

Your torso should be straight. If your torso starts to bend forward your hips tend to drop, causing you to "sit in the bucket" as we have already discussed.

> Action: Run/walk past shop windows to see if your torso is straight and make adjustments if needed.

Sag
Good technique means that the axes of your shoulders and hips remain horizontal with the ground.

"Sagging or rolling" shoulders is where your shoulders rock from side to side as you run. This causes a loss of power, and remember that poor stability means a reasonably significant loss of forward momentum.

"Sagging hips" is the effect where your hip drops to the side of the leg that is about to make contact with the ground next. As you run therefore your hips rock from side to side. This affects the smooth contact that your feet make with the ground which means your footfall will be harder and you will be braking for every stride.

Action: Use the "shop window" method and make adjustments.

Feet and knees
Feet: As you run your toes need to be pointed forward. Some runners tend to "toe out" like a duck when they run, particularly when they are fatigued. This has several effects. The first is that it can lead to groin strains, particularly if you are running a lot of hills. The second is that it affects the distance you travel per stride. A loss of something as small as half an inch per stride equates to approximately 290 yards over a half-marathon distance.

Knees: Most people's knees should track over their second and third toe counting from their big toe. Some people's knees drop further in than this (particularly women), which leads to a loss of power and can lead to knee injuries on the inside of the knee.

Action: Be aware of this and watch how your feet and knees track and make adjustments if necessary.

For those who are doing Hill Efforts (He):

Hill efforts are a very useful way to improve strength endurance and

Part 3
Week 7

therefore, indirectly, speed. The logic is based on the fact that speed for a runner in its most crude form is stride rate multiplied by strength length equals speed.

Stride Rate x Stride Length = Speed

The interesting issue in this calculation is that most people's stride rates are very similar. So one of the key characteristics that separates some runners from others is stride length. Stride length is the ability to put your foot on the ground and generate power so that you travel through the air before you touch the ground again and have to start all over. Good runners travel further through the air and can do this repeatedly for the duration of the event.

What we want to do is improve your stride length. A little like cooking, we need a recipe.

Here's what we need. We need a long smooth gentle gradient (<5%). This hill is shallow enough that your running biomechanics will be very similar to running on the flat terrain but there is enough gradient to create some resistance. Steeper hills don't provide the same opportunities, because they alter your running mechanics too much.

**Part 3
Week 7**

Most people should use a 200 yard distance, but experienced athletes can use up to 1100 yards. You run up the slope at a pace that is solid but not fast, being very careful to monitor your running form. You should not notice any real effect on the first few efforts, since the effect is only gradual. Gently jog back down after each hill effort (He), and repeat for the number of times recommended.

CHAPTER 18

WEEK EIGHT

Pacing and sports

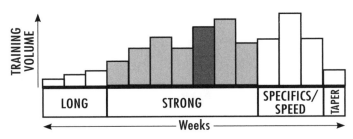

We are starting to deal with the finer points of preparing for a half-marathon. We dealt with leg speed and rhythm in the last chapter; now let's move on to pacing and running lines.

PACING—START AT THE EFFORT YOU CAN FINISH AT

A half-marathon involves balancing effort over a reasonably long duration. One of the key maxims of doing well in a half-marathon is to start at the level of effort you can finish at. Because of this, pacing is a good skill to acquire.

It's very important when you do your training runs or walks that you think about the pace you can sustain for the duration of the workout.

By running or walking too fast at the start of the event you greatly increase your chances of getting into trouble later on. The best way to avoid this is to practice pacing. Through practice you will find that you automatically lock into the correct pace on the day of the event.

In all half-marathons, pace judgement is critical. Ideally, you want to run or walk at an even pace, or even complete the second half of the event faster than the first half (called a *negative split*). Try to run or walk some of your longer workouts on out-and-back courses or circuits and try to come back slightly faster or in exactly the same time as you went out (*even split*). Never slower (*positive split*)! This is a key strategy for the event.

POOR PACING

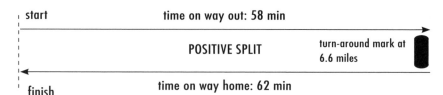

start — time on way out: 58 min

POSITIVE SPLIT — turn-around mark at 6.6 miles

finish — time on way home: 62 min

GOOD PACING (perfect!)

Part 3
Week 8

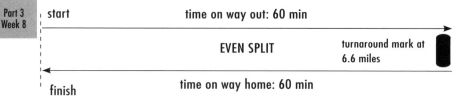

start — time on way out: 60 min

EVEN SPLIT — turnaround mark at 6.6 miles

finish — time on way home: 60 min

CONSERVATIVE BUT GOOD PACING

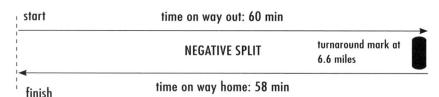

start — time on way out: 60 min

NEGATIVE SPLIT — turnaround mark at 6.6 miles

finish — time on way home: 58 min

Running lines

Never, ever run the advertised distance. Most events are measured properly down the center of where everyone will run. Obviously the trick is to cut all the corners.

In all your training, and on the day of the event, try to run or walk the shortest distance possible. Don't get too silly about this: you want to take the fastest line and sometimes the shortest line might be short but because of obstacles it is slower than a slightly wider line. Going over a hedge and through someone's garden may not be effective even if you did manage to cut the corner. Really think about the lines you are taking.

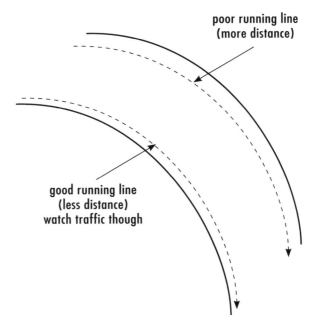

poor running line
(more distance)

good running line
(less distance)
watch traffic though

This is a good reason for training on the course prior to the event; it allows you to pre-choreograph it. You won't save huge amounts of time and distance, but why run or walk extra if you don't have to? It probably adds up to a couple of hundred yards.

Begin to incorporate pacing and running lines into your key workouts.

CHAPTER 19

WEEK NINE

Peaking control, hydration and nutrition

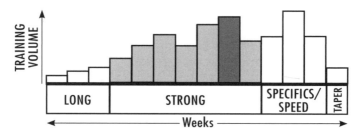

CONTROLLING PEAKING

Often as we get closer to our chosen event, it whispers in your ear "You don't have enough time to get fully ready," "You'd better hurry up, you're not going to make it" or "I can't imagine how you're going to do it." You may start to feel the pressure of what you nonchalantly committed to all those months ago.

So what happens? How do you react? Many people react by starting to crank up their training, trying to do more training, to really start to push.

Ask yourself this question: do you think most people peak too early, peak too late, or peak on time for their event? In other words, do they reach their best physical form too early, too late, or on time?

90% of the field will peak too early! How early? *Usually two to three weeks.* Which means that right now you will probably feel two or three weeks behind schedule in terms of being ready for the event.

That is normal. That's about right.

A lot of people want insurance—they want to peak before the day—but if you peak before the day you're not going to peak *on* the day. That's why it's called peaking—you can't go any higher once you are there.

Here's what you need to know to combat this "not having enough time" issue. You may feel an urge to start to push it, to wind things up or to launch headlong into the final weeks. *Don't!* Keep your training slow and go for as much strength as possible. Remember, hills, hills and . . . oh, and did I mention more hills?

With six weeks to go you're diligent in your training and no more.

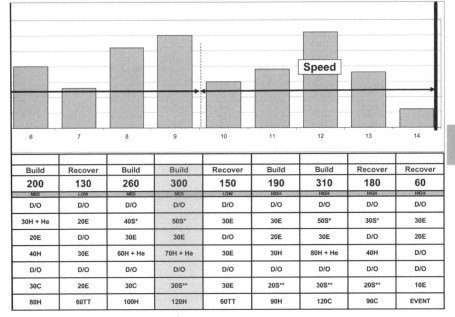

Part 3
Week 9

Build	Recover	Build	Build	Recover	Build	Build	Recover	Recover
200	**130**	**260**	**300**	**150**	**190**	**310**	**180**	**60**
MED	LOW	MED	MED	LOW	HIGH	HIGH	HIGH	HIGH
D/O	D/O	D/O	D/O	D/O	D/O	D/O	D/O	D/O
30H + He	20E	40S*	50S*	30E	30E	50S*	30S*	30E
20E	D/O	30E	30E	D/O	20E	30E	D/O	20E
40H	30E	60H + He	70H + He	30E	30H	80H + He	40H	D/O
D/O	D/O	D/O	D/O	D/O	D/O	D/O	D/O	D/O
30C	20E	30C	30S**	30E	20S**	30S**	20S**	10E
80H	60TT	100H	120H	60TT	90H	120C	90C	EVENT

Six weeks to go:
Long and strong, keep the focus and intensity down

Then you'll go into a recovery week, five weeks before the event. Slow down, catch your breath. This is like sitting on a ledge when you're climbing a mountain. You climb the cliff, then you rest on the ledge so you can continue to climb the cliff. If you don't rest on the ledge now, you'll fall off the cliff later.

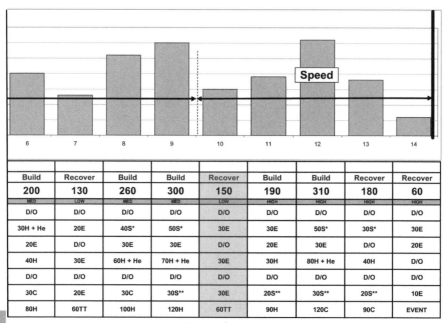

Build	Recover	Build	Build	Recover	Build	Build	Recover	Recover
200	**130**	**260**	**300**	**150**	**190**	**310**	**180**	**60**
MED	LOW	MED	MED	LOW	HIGH	HIGH	HIGH	HIGH
D/O	D/O	D/O	D/O	D/O	D/O	D/O	D/O	D/O
30H + He	20E	40S*	50S*	30E	30E	50S*	30S*	30E
20E	D/O	30E	30E	D/O	20E	30E	D/O	20E
40H	30E	60H + He	70H + He	30E	30H	80H + He	40H	D/O
D/O	D/O	D/O	D/O	D/O	D/O	D/O	D/O	D/O
30C	20E	30C	30S**	30E	20S**	30S**	20S**	10E
80H	60TT	100H	120H	60TT	90H	120C	90C	EVENT

Part 3
Week 9

**Five weeks to go:
Recovery week**

Finally, you get to four and three weeks before the event. We have already said that these are the key weeks that set up your fitness or physical ability for the event. All the training prior to this has been just to put you in the position to do these training weeks well. You want to be very focused now. Really concentrate on doing your key workouts well.

The final two weeks are your taper, which is where you freshen up for the event.

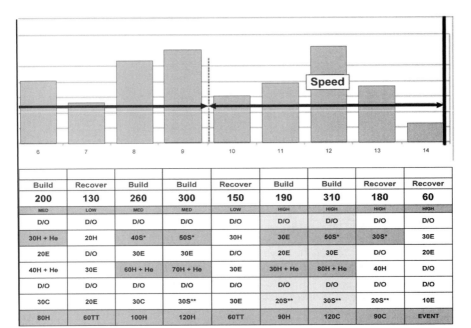

Build	Recover	Build	Build	Recover	Build	Build	Recover	Recover
200	**130**	**260**	**300**	**150**	**190**	**310**	**180**	**60**
MED	LOW	MED	MED	LOW	HIGH	HIGH	HIGH	HIGH
D/O	D/O	D/O	D/O	D/O	D/O	D/O	D/O	D/O
30H + He	20H	40S*	50S*	30H	30E	50S*	30S*	30E
20E	D/O	30E	30E	D/O	20E	30E	D/O	20E
40H + He	30E	60H + He	70H + He	30E	30H + He	80H + He	40H	D/O
D/O	D/O	D/O	D/O	D/O	D/O	D/O	D/O	D/O
30C	20E	30C	30S**	30E	20S**	30S**	20S**	10E
80H	60TT	100H	120H	60TT	90H	120C	90C	EVENT

Three and four weeks to go: Focus weeks

So, the way you treat the final six weeks of training is: diligent, rest, focused, focused, recover, recover. This will put you in the best possible condition—*peak* condition. That's what peaking is all about. By following this plan you won't overdo your training in weeks six and five before the event and will therefore avoid peaking too early.

Part 3
Week 9

HYDRATION AND NUTRITION STRATEGIES

Let's deal with your hydration and nutrition strategies before and during the event, since they have a huge impact on the result. *A 2% loss in body weight through loss of fluid will give something like a 22% loss of endurance.* So it's hugely important to make sure you have your nutrition and fluids taken care of.

We need to look at two areas: energy in the muscles and fluid in the tank. You need to practice these hydration and nutrition strategies in your longer workouts from now until event day so you have this area locked down.

Practice for the night before

Energy in the muscles:
Carbohydrate is turned into glycogen in the body and glycogen is what makes your legs work. It's very important that you have tons of glycogen in your legs on the day of the event to avoid prematurely fatiguing and the only way to do that is to do what is called *carbohydrate loading*.

To do this, you need to have high-carbohydrate meals two to three days before and the night before the event. That means lots of rice, pasta, bread, potatoes—that sort of thing. You don't eat *more* food, you just need to have a greater proportion of carbohydrates.

Electrolytes in the muscles:
You want to be drinking fruit juices or fluids that contain electrolytes (which is a fancy way of saying sodium, or salt and potassium). These electrolytes are important because they allow your muscles to function correctly so you don't get cramping, and at worst low sodium/potassium levels on the day.

Therefore, you want to make sure that you hydrate a little bit more than you usually would, using fruit juices or drinks which will replace the sodium and potassium being lost in training. If you just drink water you flush all the electrolytes out of your body, which will raise your chances of cramping. There are many commercial carbohydrate and electrolyte replacement drinks available in the fridge at your corner store or supermarket.

Hydration and urine color:
Please excuse me for talking about this, but it is a necessity for half-marathon running!

On the night before and on the morning of the event your urine should be clear. This indicates you're well hydrated. When your urine has a yellow color that means it's very concentrated—and this is not good.

If you drink a lot of fluids your urine becomes more diluted, hence it becomes more clear. So a clear urine color the night before is very important to indicate whether you're adequately hydrated. I'm sure you're not normally interested in the color of your urine, but in this case it's probably a good idea.

If you are taking multivitamins they will cause the urine color to remain yellow. In this case, you will know that you are well hydrated if you are urinating copiously the night before the event. In fact, it should be hard to sit down for more than about two hours.

Practice for event morning

Event morning, or in the morning before your long training runs or walks, have a standard breakfast. Don't have anything complicated—just a standard breakfast. Make sure it's not too high in fiber though, because too much fiber can cause runner's diarrhea. Have breakfast between two and three hours before your workout (ideally three hours before if you can realistically do it).

Practice for during the event

During the event, and during your long training sessions, you want to be drinking two to three mouthfuls of a carbohydrate–electrolyte replacement drink every 15 minutes, a little bit less on a cold day, a little bit more if it's hot. These pre-mixed drinks are available at almost any café, service station or corner store. They contain a 7% solution of carbohydrates plus electrolytes.

Part 3
Week 9

If you drink every 15 minutes you will keep your energy levels stable and have a much more successful long run or walk, faster recovery and a much more successful event.

It is only necessary to practice event hydration on your long training sessions. For your mid-week runs and walks that are less than 60 minutes in duration, just hydrate with water.

On event day you'll get your hydration either from the aid stations, or you may decide to carry your own fluid in a fluid backpack or fluid belt. These are available in most sporting goods stores and are a great investment. If you choose to use one of these in the event you will need to practice carrying your fluid this way on all your long training sessions from this point on.

If you are going to use aid stations, obviously you can't easily set up "practice" aid stations for your long practice runs, so stashing fluid bottles along your intended course before you start is usually the way to go. Start practicing!

CHAPTER 20

WEEK TEN

The 80/20 rule, the push and gadgets

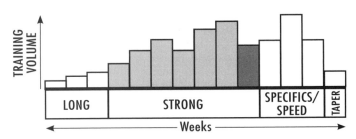

THE 80/20 RULE

At this point the 80/20 rule becomes very important. You are now coming into the key weeks of your program. To recap: the 80/20 rule, when applied to training, means that 20% of the workouts you do will have an 80% effect on how you perform in the final event.

The "vital few" are color-coded in the programs for you, but just for the record, the most important workouts are time trials (if you have them in your program) followed by your longest workout on the course, followed by your longest workouts. Speed workouts follow but are not as valuable.

This means that at this point in the program, week ten, you need to be more alert to making sure you are ready for the key 80/20 workouts coming up. You have reached a point where the workouts *with* the most impact are being done at the point in your program that *has* most impact, doubling their value.

Try to make sure you are "fresh" enough to do these key workouts well (particularly time trials and course workouts).

THE PUSH

Remember that the next two weeks are your focus weeks. These weeks have more impact, from a training standpoint, on your event than any other weeks. The other weeks were trained just to put you in a position to do these two weeks well. This does not mean that you want to overdo the next few weeks, but it does mean you should rest up this week and be gentle on your workouts so that you go into the following weeks fresh enough to train well and get the most out of your training.

GADGETS

There are two very convenient gadgets that you may want to purchase at this point.

↓   Heart rate monitors

↓   Speedometer devices

Heart Rate Monitors:

Heart rate monitors measure how often your heart beats. The harder you work, the higher the heart rate and the slower you go, the lower your heart rate. So a heart rate monitor is like a rev counter giving you an idea of your effort at any given time.

Here is an indication of how the heart rates apply to your training. Most heart monitors allow you to enter your age so that they can give you a percentage of your maximum heart rate, which is very similar to percentage effort as opposed to the raw heart rate numbers.

Code	Description	Heart Rate (as % of Maximum HR)
E	Easy	60 – 75%
H	Hills	60 – 75% most of the time (up to 80% on hills)

C	Course	60 – 75%
He	Hill Efforts	70 – 80% during the effort (60 – 70% jogging back down)
TT	Time Trial	usually 75 – 85%
S*	Speed 1	usually 75 – 85% (NO FASTER!)
S**	Speed 2	85 – 95%
S	Speed	usually 75 – 85% (NO FASTER!)
R	Run	60 – 75% (ideally closer to 60% initially)
W	Walk	50 – 65%
RW	Run Walk	A combination of the above

If you don't have a heart rate monitor that expresses heart rate as a percentage of maximum heart rate, try the following calculation, which works for most people.

First determine maximum predicted heart rate and then use the percentages in the above table to determine the actual raw heart rate ranges.

Maximum Predicted Heart rate

Males: 220 minus your age

Females: 226 minus your age

e.g. 220 – 35yrs = 185

185 x 60% = 111

185 x 75% = 138

Part 3
Week 10

This will not work for everyone, so try to match your heart rate percentages with the equal percentage effort. For example, you might find to match your percentage effort with the heart rate percentages you might need to add 10 to all of your calculations.

Speedometers

In recent times running speedometers have become available. The speeds are determined through GPS or through accelerometers in foot pods worn on the shoe laces of your running shoes.

This has probably been the biggest running innovation in the last 20 years! The reason for this is that you can accurately pace yourself correctly. In week eight we discussed pacing and how it was important to running/ walking at your best. You needed to even or negative split your runs/walks and this was a little difficult as you were doing this by "feel," which gets even harder to get right when all the distractions of the event hype occur on the "big day." With a running speedometer you determine what you think is the correct speed in your pacing practice and time trials and then all you have to do on the day is run/walk to the correct speed shown on the device on average, taking into account the ups and downs of the terrain. This means that you will have perfect pacing!

Part 3
Week 10

CHAPTER 21

WEEK ELEVEN

The need for speed

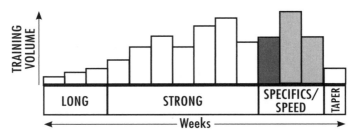

Your body should now be shown what speed it's going to be traveling at on event day. It should also be trained for the conditions you will encounter: the terrain or, better still, the actual course. Problems usually occur only if you get a surprise or have not prepared for an aspect of the event.

Of course, you may choose not to do any speed work. A lot of the training programs in this book do not have speed work in them. *But you must be ready for the course.*

SPEED

The speed work that you do in training should be *at exactly the speed you do in the event*. It should be no different. Don't get sucked in to thinking faster is better. It only leads to trouble.

You need to show your body exactly what's going to happen on the day, so this means showing your body the right speed. In other words, leave your testosterone at home. Remember there are no medals, no certificates and no prizes given out in training.

In addition, training too fast will only teach you to go out much too fast on the day of the event, and that's not helpful—remember pacing, and starting at the effort you can finish at.

If you constantly train too fast, the only time your body will experience the speed that you will run or walk on the day of the event is on the day of the event, and this is not a good recipe for a good day!

If you choose to do speed work, estimate a speed that you feel you can cope with and train specifically at that pace. Running terminology usually describes speed in minutes taken to run or walk a mile. So you might train yourself to run at 9½ minutes per mile.

You need to train your ability to know this by feel and set yourself up to be able to consistently maintain it. Don't worry too much about the ups and downs of the course, as the slower speed taken to go up the hills is usually cancelled out by the speed taken to come down them.

Work out what perceived effort is required to maintain your chosen speed, then try to keep the effort the same and let the speed take care of itself.

**Part 3
Week 11**

By the time you turn up on event day you want to have repeatedly shown your body the speed it needs to go at. It should be second nature and you should feel confident that it can be maintained for the full duration of the event.

If your program contains speed work, the notes will contain information about how much and what types of speed work you should do.

SPECIFICS

Course

If you can, train on the course, or something very similar to it, several times. It doesn't have to be every day, but often enough so your body knows what to expect on event day. Even driving over the course the day before is better than going in cold.

Knowing the course makes a big difference. If I set you a 3 mile run or walk at event pace on a course you know, and a 3 mile run or walk at event pace on a course you don't know, which one would you go faster on?

You guessed it: *the one that you know*. Why? Because you are better able to judge your pace and progress. You know exactly where you are. You know how to spread your energy out over the whole event.

So, make sure you know the course as well as you possibly can. Know the corners, the hills, the turns, where the shade is, and where the wind might be strongest. Know the faster lines (the lines you are going to run or walk) and the slower lines (the lines you don't want to run/walk).

In training, start thinking: "Take the fastest line." Focus on going the quickest and most economical way from point A to point B. If you go around a corner, go around the inside, not the outside (see "Running lines," page 103).

Environmental conditions

Another aspect of the race to simulate is the time of day you will do the half-marathon. At least once in training, do your workout at the same time, and on the same day of the week, as the event will be held. Also, practice your pre-event routine, even if it means getting up at 3:30 a.m.! That way you will know what the temperature is going to be like, and you will find out whether or not you need to wear a tracksuit before the start. You will also have a better idea of how much time you need to get ready for the event.

Part 3
Week 11

Other details

Also practice what you will drink during the event (find out what the sponsored event fluid is) so you're used to it, and any other specifics that the event requires.

No changes

You should not make any changes to shoes, socks or event clothing after this point. Everything should be tried and true well before the event. No changes, no surprises.

A RECAP OF THE FUNDAMENTAL LAWS OF TRAINING

Law one: the training program
Take the sport, break it into parts, train each part and slowly put it back together again as you get closer and closer to the main event, so your body knows exactly what it's going to be doing. Show your body the sport, how to do the sport well, how far it will go, how much muscular effort is required, how fast it will go, what the details are and where it will do all this.

Law two: the training
Training in its simplest sense is: Mimic what will happen on the day, and when you can't, stop!

If you follow these two laws, by the time you show up on event day it will be very, very hard to get anything wrong.

Through training you show your body . . .

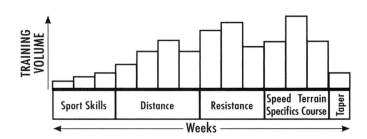

CHAPTER 22

WEEK TWELVE

Controlling technique

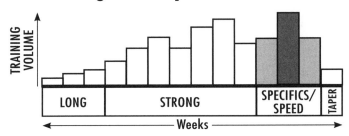

TECHNIQUE—ONE MORE TIME

There is one last point to mention about technique. So far we have covered the theory in terms of how running/walking works, and you have practiced it. The discussion of technique has been designed to help cover the little things that might help you to be more comfortable, less injured and a bit faster.

What we now want to talk about is the other key area, which is not so much about getting faster but about not slowing down.

Getting faster is only important if you don't slow down and, believe it or not, this is a big part of half-marathon running and walking. As we have said before, most people start too fast and "blow up."

So how does technique affect this?

As you fatigue in an event, you physically begin to deteriorate but you also begin to technically deteriorate. You may have stood at the end of a half-marathon before and seen all the variously strange gaits and body angles of people crossing the line. The trick is that you can't really control how you physically deteriorate except for correct pacing, but you can have a huge effect on how you technically deteriorate to the point that you don't deteriorate technique-wise at all.

The first half of the event should be fine in terms of technique; it's in the second half that things can start to become harder and unravel. So now that you have practiced your technique and more importantly are aware of how your body should be operating, you now monitor your technique as you begin to tire. Any areas that have deteriorated need to be modified to keep you efficient, comfortable and fast to the end of the event.

Often it's the third quarter where things most need to be pulled back into line.

During your long runs/walks (and particularly your time trials if you have them) try to focus on maintaining your form towards the end of the workout to practice this for the "big day."

Going into Taper
Remember that you can give this week a little more effort because things will get easier from here on in your training. Next week you move into your taper, which means you move from the training phase of your program into the maintaining and freshening phase.

CHAPTER 23

WEEK THIRTEEN

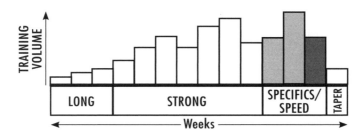

The taper

With seven to ten days to go, we now move into the taper.

All the training you have done so far has been to boost your performance. In this final phase of your training program you are focusing on using recovery to boost your performance as you freshen up from the cumulative fatigue of training.

You need to:
- physically recover
- mentally recover
- wake up the body

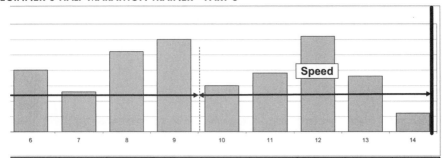

Build	Recover	Build	Build	Recover	Build	Build	Recover	Recover
200	**130**	**260**	**300**	**150**	**190**	**310**	**180**	**60**
MED	LOW	MED	MED	LOW	HIGH	HIGH	HIGH	HIGH
D/O	D/O	D/O	D/O	D/O	D/O	D/O	D/O	D/O
30H + He	20E	40S*	50S*	30E	30E	50S*	30S*	30E
20E	D/O	30E	30E	D/O	20E	30E	D/O	20E
40H	30E	60H + He	70H + He	30E	30H	80H + He	40H	D/O
D/O	D/O	D/O	D/O	D/O	D/O	D/O	D/O	D/O
30C	20E	30C	30S**	30E	20S**	30S**	20S**	10E
80H	60TT	100H	120H	60TT	90H	120C	90C	EVENT

two and one week to go:
Taper/recovery

PHYSICAL RECOVERY

In these last few weeks, you will notice that the lengths of the workouts are steadily dropping. This is to make sure that your workouts from here on do not overly tire you. This allows you to physically "power up": your performance should go up another 2 to 5% during this period. (A little secret though: you won't actually feel powered up until you start the event.) However, you do still need to keep your training intensity up to maintain the training you have done.

Part 3
Week 13

MENTAL RECOVERY

You also need to mentally power up.

During your training you've gotten up early in the morning, gone to work, picked something up at lunchtime, worked hard all day, picked up some groceries on the way home . . . and then you've gone training. And then, after training, you've cooked dinner, washed the dishes, done a few chores and, finally, gone to bed.

And the next day . . . well, I'm sure you've heard of *Groundhog Day*.

You need to understand that this event is not only about physical endurance. It's also about mental endurance. Therefore, from a mental viewpoint, as the event gets close, you need to start storing some mental energy.

How do you do that? Very simply.

Use distractions that you enjoy and that naturally relax you, like going to the movies, reading a book, going out to dinner, making or listening to music, or walking the dog, to allow you to step away from the things in life that use up your willpower and mental effort. You don't want to think about the event every minute of every hour for the next 14 days.

WAKING UP THE BODY

At the same time as we are physically powering up, we also need to wake the body up.

Why do we do this? Let me illustrate with a common experience. Many of us work five days in a row, then have the weekend off. When you start back at work on Monday, you often feel like you've got "Monday-morning-itis."

Essentially, you've disrupted your circadian rhythms (the body's 24-hour sleeping, waking and breakfast, lunch and dinner cycles) during the weekend. When you get up early and go back to work on Monday, you've got what could be described as a mild form of jet lag.

How does this relate to the event? Well, when you get up the day before the event, chances are you'll be thinking: "I can hardly get out of bed. I have no idea how I'm going to do a half-marathon tomorrow." This is probably because you didn't train the day before and you are "out of sync."

If you have a day off the day before the event, you'll have your "Monday morning-itis" during the event. End result? You lack energy, can't get going, and feel blah.

To avoid the blahs, you have a day off *two days before the event*. Then you exercise the day before the event to get back in sync with your circadian rhythms.

If you do this, you'll be a few percent better on the day than you've been at any part of your training program. This is because everything you've done so far has been done while you've been "loaded up" on training. Every time you've trained, it's always been after another training session. Race day will be the only time where you actually do some exercise fully "unloaded" of cumulative fatigue. Trust me, this makes a huge difference.

Other issues

Making changes
As I said in the previous chapter, do not make any changes to your shoes, socks, event clothing or event nutrition and hydration. Everything should be tried and true. No changes, no surprises.

Travel
If the event you are training for is being held somewhere else, in another city, for example, you should aim to be at the location at least two nights before event day. This allows you to have your final training session on, and get to know, the course.

Event/Race vs. long training day

The word "race" means many things to many people. But if it means "pain," "hurting," or "competing" to you, and these are not helpful as you prepare for the event, you might want to think about it in a different way.

For example, thinking of the event as "a long training day" may be less threatening or scary. If you think this way, you may find it a lot easier to control the event and yourself.

Of course, if you're a first-timer, don't even think about "racing." It's not a race. You're not showing up to race somebody, you're showing up *to complete an event*.

**Part 3
Week 13**

Going for a time
For you first-timers, time is not on your side. Time is the dirtiest word in the first-time half-marathoner's dictionary.

You've never done a half-marathon before. So how do you have any idea how long it will take you? *You don't!*

Too often first-timers say they are going to do this time, or that time. All this does is create pressure.

Remember, *the only half-marathon in which you will never have any time pressure is your first one.* So don't waste that chance—don't put yourself under that sort of pressure.

I have seen people who have dreamed of doing a half-marathon for years and years. They finally get to the event, they complete the event, they step across the line, and at the one moment when they should be celebrating they go, "Oh, that's not very fast." Sadly, this is how to be a winner and a loser at exactly the same time!

So, if somebody asks you, "What time are you going to do?" your answer is: "I'm going to finish some time in daylight." Which is a polite way of saying, "Don't ask me a dumb question."

Don't get sucked in to predicting your time. Enjoy the event, celebrate at the finish, but don't race the clock.

So this week the program is starting to take care of your physical recovery. You now need to work on the mental recovery aspect.

CHAPTER 24

WEEK FOURTEEN—Read on the Monday before the event!

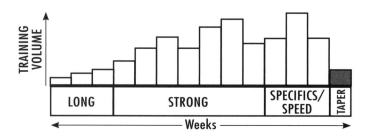

The final countdown

SLEEP

The sleep you get from three days before the event is more important than the sleep you get the night before. Try to set up these evenings so you are pretty relaxed but also distracted, so the event is not at the forefront of your mind, keeping you awake.

Phantom pains

It is quite common this close to the event to get "phantom pains." These are little pains that suddenly appear out of nowhere in the last few days. The reason this happens is that your body starts to become super-sensitive. It will notice aches and pains that you have not noticed before. The ankle you hurt six weeks ago suddenly starts to hurt again. In fact, the pain never went away; you have just suddenly noticed it again because you are a little more sensitive.

Don't let this psych you out; phantom pains affect about 50% of people doing events and they have a 99.9% chance of disappearing on the day, despite how concerning and "real" they might feel to you right now. Don't sweat it. If you are really worried, check with a doctor as soon as you can to allay your fears.

Nutrition

With three days to go you should start carbohydrate loading. This means eating more pasta, potatoes, rice and bread. You do not need to eat more food; you just need to eat more carbohydrates for breakfast, lunch and dinner. As mentioned in Chapter 16, this is important because carbohydrates turn into glycogen, and glycogen fuels the legs. We've already said that your legs are the limiting factor in a half-marathon, so if you can carbohydrate load, it's going to make a big difference.

The intimidation factor

You need to be mentally prepared for this. Once you arrive in the event environment you may think that everyone else looks like a professional athlete, with all the gear. This can be a little intimidating, but the trick is to understand that a lot of these people have all the gear and no ideas, and that you are not the only person who feels like this. Just about *everyone* feels like this to some extent. Join the club! Even most of the athletes aiming to do well can feel it. (In fact, even the spectators can feel it and they aren't even participating!) It's OK: you are not the odd one out, so don't sweat it.

Get an overview of the course

If you haven't already, go over the course to get a feel for it. If you can, drive over the course and try to gain an understanding of what it's like. Stop often and get out and really have a good look. You might be interested in getting a feel for the following:

Part 3
Week 14

- road surface and pot-holes
- hill gradients
- landmarks to gauge distances and your progress.

If you can, go over the course with someone who is experienced at looking at a course, like a coach, or take someone who has done the event before and get them to explain it.

THE DAY BEFORE

Do your final workout

Go out and do your final "wake-up" workout. As you exercise, focus on trying to establish the effort and rhythm you want to maintain the following day. This helps you to warm up and pre-set the key issues.

Try to do this workout on the course.

Prepare your gear

Always prepare your gear the day before the event. If you rush around trying to find your gear on the morning of the event you will discover that most of the marbles have dropped out of your head and you'll forget something important like . . . your running shoes.

Pin your event number on your running shirt. Make sure the pins aren't going to cause chafing and that it doesn't get in the way. Position it so you don't even know it's there.

Pack your "event bag" so that it contains everything you need:
- Vaseline
- sunblock
- warm clothing for after the event
- a drink to sip on going to the start
- money

Get a weather forecast

Around noon, check the weather forecast for the following day so you know what you are in for.

The key things to know, in order of priority, are:
- which way the wind will be blowing (will it make some parts of the course harder?)
- how hard the wind will be blowing
- whether it is likely to rain
- how hot or cold it will be.

In the afternoon, relax. Do things that allow you to switch off.

Dinner

That night, have a normal-sized carbohydrate meal. Do not have too much—otherwise, you will have difficulty sleeping.

Have fruit juice or some fluid that contains electrolytes, rather than water, with your meal, to maintain high electrolyte levels.

If you do not take multivitamins, your urine color should be clear that evening. If you do take multivitamins, your urine color will remain yellow, but you should need to go to the bathroom a number of times indicating that you are well hydrated.

Bedtime

- Set your alarms (set multiple alarms, on multiple clocks and watches)
- Lay out all your gear
- Set up tomorrow's breakfast (all within easy reach)
- Make sure there's enough gas in the car (and go get some if you need to)
- Don't go to bed early.

If you go to bed at 7 you will be lying in bed awake until 11. Most people go to sleep one to two hours later than normal on the night before the event.

The amount of sleep you get the night before does not matter. If you are lying in bed and have worked out that there are exactly 256 tiles on the ceiling, get up and do something that relaxes you. Do not lie in bed waiting for the dawn.

- Finally, drift off to sleep.

Part 3
Week 14

CHAPTER 25

WEEK FOURTEEN—Read on the Wednesday before the event!

A run-down of event day

This chapter covers everythng you need to know and think about now and on event day.

2½ TO 3½ HOURS BEFORE START TIME

You wake to the sound of your first alarm going off. Then the second alarm, then the third. You are irritated a few minutes later by the fourth alarm going off. You're awake, it is all going by plan so far!

You want to get up about 2½ to 3½ hours before the event starts. This gives your body enough time to wake up. It also gives you enough time to do everything you need to do in an unhurried manner, including checking your gear. Feeling rushed before an event is a common reason for athletes to have a poor start.

The first thing to do is put on the gear you will wear for the event, put on your tracksuit (if you need one) over the top of that, then go and have some breakfast. Another good reason for the early start is that you want enough time to digest breakfast and have your morning "constitutional" at home—standing in a line of 20 people outside a smelly port-a-potty should be avoided if at all possible.

You want your breakfast to be low in fiber. This means white bread, not whole wheat, and cornflakes rather than granola or muesli. Bananas are also good, as is a cup of fruit juice. You should have been practicing your event-morning breakfast for the last six weeks.

Take a bottle of water or electrolyte drink to sip in the car on the way to the event.

1 to 1½ hours before start time

Going to and arriving at the event

You want to arrive at the event *about an hour before start time*. This means leaving home earlier than you would normally. Why? Well, when you get to within about 1 mile of the start you'll discover that it's rush hour. It may take you 20 minutes to move 550 yards. So be prepared for that.

Once you've parked your car, or gotten off the bus or ferry, go and take a look at the start area, just to familiarize yourself with where you need to be.

To deal with the pressure, you need to focus on you and your own long training day. Don't let the chaos around you infiltrate your thinking. No one else exists. There are going to be a few thousand other people doing exactly the same thing, at exactly the same time, at exactly the same place as you. But that's just a coincidence. When the gun goes off you will do your own thing.

Focus on yourself. Don't worry about what others are doing in their warm-up, what they are wearing, what shoes they've got on, or whether they are built for speed or comfort. Focus on your own effort, rhythm and pace.

If you are going to race the event, go for a five to seven minute run about 25 to 30 minutes before the start time. Try and do about three one-minute efforts at what you think your event pace will be (no faster!), with easy jogs in between to allow your body to recover.

If your goal is to complete the event, just go for a five to ten minute walk or run in your tracksuit with about 25 minutes to go. Then take your tracksuit off, give it to your friends or family or put it in your support bag (which will be taken to the finish line by the event organizers), and make

Part 3
Week 14

131

your way down to the start.

If you think the weather might be cold it's a good idea to wear an old t-shirt or sweatshirt over the top of your event gear to stay warm, then discard it just before the gun (somebody will pick it up). A plastic garbage bag with armholes and a hole cut out for your head is good as a disposable rain coat if you think it is going to rain (just make sure you don't sweat too much in it and get chilled when you take the bag off just before the start).

To avoid chafing, put Vaseline (or another product you've found) between your thighs and under your armpits. Guys, if it's a cold day you may also want to put Band-Aids over your nipples, since they too can chafe and, ultimately, bleed. This is painful and will make the event less enjoyable, plus your finisher's photo will not be a Rembrandt!

Ten minutes before start time

Make your way to the starting line.

If you are a first-timer, just slot yourself in where you feel comfortable. If you know your predicted time, do your best to position yourself among runners of the same level of ability, so you don't get stuck behind slower runners at the start and you can pace yourself with runners with the same speed. Often there are signs up indicating predicted finishing times—1:30, 1:45, and so on—so it's just a matter of standing in that particular area.

However, if there are no signs, or people seem to be ignoring them, you just have to have a look around at everyone, guess what their ability level might be, and slot yourself in somewhere. Often at the front of your predicted finish-time group is good.

At this point, especially if you are a first-timer, you may be asking yourself, "What am I doing here?" Well, just remember, around 14 weeks earlier, you had a good reason for wanting to complete this event. *Today is just a long training day, not a race.* Just relax and enjoy it.

These thoughts will help you control the stress and the event.

Part 3
Week 14

FIVE MINUTES BEFORE START TIME

Remember pace and rhythm

The secret to successfully completing any endurance event is to get your pacing right. We are all familiar with the fable about the tortoise and the hare. On the day, slow and steady won the race for the tortoise. You don't have to aim for slow, but do aim for steady.

If you remember one thing about event day, remember this: *start at a pace or effort that you believe you can finish at.*

The most efficient way to exercise over a long period of time is to have an even or consistent effort for the first 99% of the distance. If you start too quickly, you are likely to struggle in the second half of the event. Believe me, this is not fun. And if you start *way* too quickly, you risk not finishing at all.

So, start at a pace you can finish at . . . and leave the hares to it.

I now want you to imagine this: imagine the atmosphere . . . imagine the tension . . .

There are thousands of people milling around. The air is seriously amped. There is a lot of nervous energy being generated.

With about 25 minutes to go, you do a bit of a warm-up for five minutes, take off your tracksuit, and pack it in your bag.

With about ten minutes to go, you make your way down to the start line. You notice people are either jiggling around on the spot, talking nervously or looking seriously amped.

With about five minutes to go, you listen to the final briefing. With about two minutes to go, you are put in the starter's hands.

The countdown begins: 10, 9, 8 . . .

Bang! The gun goes off.

How do you think most of the people will react? Right! They go off at 900,000,000 miles an hour (or faster than the speed of light!). And the event goes, "Got ya!"

Part 3
Week 14

You see, the event tries to wind you up, like a spring, in the last hour before the start. It hopes you will charge off at, well, 900,000,000 miles an hour (above light speed).

The start is almost the event's last throw of the dice to defeat you. This is when you need to show the event that *you are in control.*

You must be disciplined. Remember, you must start at a pace you can finish at. Don't join the headless chicken brigade (about 80% of the field!).

If you start with "a long training day," you end up with a race. If you start with a race, you often end up with a barbecue, and you're the one who gets cooked!

Now, this is what you need to do:

Bang! The gun goes off.
- Try to relax as much as possible.
- Think relax, rhythm, pace. You should have practiced rhythm and pace or effort a number of times so you can simply lock in on it.
- Try to get into your own space. Don't get distracted by anybody else. The event's going to be saying to you: "Look at that person, look at that person, look at that person."
- Focus on yourself, relax, and get into a rhythm and pace as soon as you can. This may take five or ten minutes unless you've done plenty of event-pace specific practice.

AID STATIONS AND DEMONS

You should drink at every aid station unless you've practiced with and are wearing some sort of drinking system like a backpack or a bottle belt. At every aid station, pick up a cup of carbohydrate drink and a cup of water. As you pick up the cups, pinch the tops so you can funnel the liquid into your mouth without spilling too much of it.

If the temperature is moderate you'll need to drink about three mouthfuls at each aid station (two carbohydrate/electrolyte drink and one water early on; two water and one carbohydrate/electrolyte later). Note that your body will probably want to drink more carbohydrate early in the event and more water late in the event.

Part 3
Week 14

134

After your three mouthfuls—glug, glug, glug—throw the cups away, even if they're half full. They will be picked up by volunteers.

If you're racing, grab your cups, drink, and keep running. Don't be surprised if you cough and splutter a little bit—it's not easy to drink when moving fast.

If you're walking, just walk—don't even break step!

If you're not racing, go into a fast walk as you enter the aid station, pick up the cups—glug, glug, glug—and then start running again.

The reason you walk fast at the aid stations is to try to keep your rhythm. If you break rhythm it can hurt your legs and waste energy as you try to get back up to speed.

But beware the demons . . .

Aid-station demons are the little guys who sit on your shoulder and say terrible things to you each time you get to an aid station.

At the first aid station the little demon says, "You should go into a fast walk and pick up those drinks." You think, "That's OK, no problem with that."

At the second aid station the little demon will say to you, "Ah, but you need to catch your breath first. Walk into the aid station and pick up your drinks and then run out the other side." And you think, "That's fair, I can totally understand that."

Then at the third aid station the little demon says to you, "Boy, those drinks are important. You need to walk out the other side."

Before you know it, you are walking . . . and the more you walk, the more you want to walk.

So, try to keep your rhythm through the aid stations, and don't let the "demons" get you.

Step by step

The half-marathon may be 13.1 miles but it's also just a whole lot of single steps (or tasks) linked together.

**Part 3
Week 14**

When the gun goes off, the first thing you do is run 220 yards along the road. Then you might turn right. And then, soon, you might turn left . . . and so on. The event is just a series of tasks joined together.

If you recall, I said that training is simply showing your body what happens on the day. This is so the body is good at all the tasks it needs to be good at in order to complete the event.

The reason that you can drive a car so easily now is that you've practiced all the driving tasks over and over again. It's become automatic. Remember when you began driving? It probably felt very clumsy—your body and mind had not yet practiced all the tasks sufficiently to make it smooth and efficient.

The same is true with doing this event. By practicing all the tasks, and by knowing the course, you will find that on event day everything becomes automatic. Just another day at the office!

For example, you know that on this section you'll be running or walking into a headwind, so you might drop in behind somebody. At another point you might know you'll be running or walking with a tailwind so, since it's a hot day, you need to put some water over your head.

You want to show up on the day and have the whole event programmed in, so all that's left to do is to run the program.

This is really important. Training is not just about going out for a run or a walk; it's about going out and practicing all the aspects that will make up the event.

Either you control the event, or the event controls you. If it's neutral territory, it gets a whole lot easier for the event to start to control you. But if you know the course like you know your living room, it's going to be really hard for the event to do anything to you.

WHEN IS HALFWAY NOT HALFWAY?

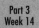
Part 3
Week 14

OK, the event has tried to stop you getting to the starting line, it's given you little pains or problems, and it's made you sick for a week so you've missed training. But here you are, 3 miles into it . . . you've beaten the event, right?
Not yet!

The best description of a half-marathon is that it's a 9 mile warm-up and a 4 mile running race (if you are running the event). In other words, halfway is not 6.5 miles.

In terms of effort it's the final 4 miles that counts. At the 9 mile point the event will try to ambush you. It will say, "Surprise, I'm taking over."

Your answer to that is, "Bring it on. I've been waiting for you all day." You expected this; that's why you started at a pace you could finish at.

The event will then say, "Yeah, you might have been waiting for this all day, but if you feel tired now, imagine trying to keep going for another 4 miles. You can't do that."

Fortunately, we know that within 1.5 or 2 miles of the finish line you will start to feel better. Your energy and enthusiasm will increase as you start to get excited about finishing.

So it's not a whole 4 miles; it's only about 2 miles of gritting your teeth before things get better again!

If you're planning to race the event you should also know this: the point when you think you've started to slow down, and the point you *actually* slow down, are often quite different.

For the first 9 miles your pace is almost locked in—you just roll on, without having to concentrate too hard to maintain your pace. But at 9 miles, as you start to tire, you'll think, "Oh my gosh, I'm starting to slow down." *Don't worry.*

We know that you will probably hold your speed for another 2.4–3 miles, even if it doesn't feel like it. So maintain your effort, stay focused on your goal and let your preparation get you home.

Having said that, the last 3 or 4 miles is where your understanding of the course—the turns, landmarks—will really pay dividends.

Part 3
Week 14

CROSSING THE LINE

There tend to be two types of people who enter half-marathons. The first is the "completer." This is the person who said at the beginning, "I just want to complete this." Please don't be a "completer" who, five minutes after finishing, is saying, "Oh, I'm really unhappy with my time."

If you aim to complete, then complete. That's it. You've achieved your goal. Enjoy the moment. Embrace it. Squeeze it. Be happy!

If you're more experienced and aiming for a time—a "competer"—that's a little bit different. But you still need to keep your focus on the tasks—on what you need to do to achieve your time (e.g. get to the start early, warm up, seed yourself correctly, start at a pace you can maintain to the finish, get into your rhythm quickly, run the fastest lines, etc).

The most successful athletes in the world understand this. They have a goal of winning, or setting a time (the outcome), but once that goal is set, they shift their focus to what is needed to produce a great performance (the process).

IMMEDIATELY AFTER YOU CROSS THE LINE

So you've crossed the line—but you still have one last set of tasks to perform. First, if you do not feel good medically—which is very, very rare—see a medic at the finish line immediately, as they can help you sort things out. You also will want something to eat and drink.

Your body will super-compensate for the energy you take in at this point in terms of recovering lost energy. A carbohydrate/electrolyte replacement drink or fruit juice is a good fluid option. Eat something that your body wants to eat or craves right now. Try to have what your body wants rather than deciding what it needs. Stretch if you feel like it and have a light recovery massage if you can.

This is designed to ensure that:
- You don't fall asleep in your food tonight through lack of energy.
- You can work the next day rather than sitting, drooling, at your desk, staring blankly at your computer screen.
- You can walk around normally the next day, rather than having that sore/stiff-legged "cowboy" walk that often occurs.

THE NEXT DAY

Go for a short, gentle walk to loosen up your legs. Include a stop at a café halfway if you have the time. If your legs are particularly sore, try to move around at regular intervals during the day to keep your legs from stiffening up too much.

THE WEEKS FOLLOWING THE EVENT

Have an off-season. It usually takes about three to six weeks to physically and mentally recover (you'll think you've recovered in a week but you would be wrong). Ideally you should keep doing a little bit of training in the week or so after the event—your body hates sudden changes which throw it off, so a little bit of training is often good. One or two 20-minute runs or walks would be good.

Part 3
Week 14

What did you achieve?

First, let's look at the health aspects.

Remember the attitude study? You will have pushed back the boundaries. You'll have a young attitude; you'll be younger mentally. You'll probably live longer because of it.

Then there was the Harvard Study. You'll age more slowly; you'll be young for your age. You'll be young physically.

Furthermore, you'll have a huge improvement in your health profile. You'll have a 31% reduction in your risk of cancer, and a 43% reduction in your risk of heart disease. That is huge.

On top of that, the corporate business studies show this is not a con. We know it works.

The numerous studies on achievement say that most people self-limit. You won't. You will experience *everything*.

You've had an adventure.

And all of this will be for 1.5% of your time. What a win!

You have learned lots about exercise and training and you have completed a really cool event. Hopefully you completed well and I bet you had some fun along the way.

What next?

What next, you ask? Do the event again for a faster time, or choose a new goal that inspires you.

If you choose to do the half-marathon again, go back to the start of this book and select a slightly higher-level training program. Work on the areas you felt weaker in.

If you choose a new goal, remember: you will be surprised at what you can do if you give yourself a chance.

Whether you are returning to do another half-marathon or off on a new quest, don't forget that Performance Lab's skilled staff have a range of services including books and more advanced training programs to help you explore, conquer and enjoy your training.

And finally . . .

If you have any stories to tell, tricks you've learned that you'd like to pass on to others or event reports, please send them to us via *www.performancelab.co.nz*—we'd like to hear from you.

Live long and perspire!—Jon

Epilogue

ACKNOWLEDGMENTS

This book was written in all sorts of places: New Zealand, Dubai Airport, Melbourne Airport, Heathrow Airport and Valencia. It is a real testament to others who helped put this together, because it required editing and proofing by people in different parts of the world.

Brett Reid was the ghost writer and, as usual, did a fantastic job. Denise Matthews did a lot of the proofing and coordination and, as usual, had everything running like clockwork; Kerri McMaster held things together.

Thanks also to Margaret Sinclair, my editor from Random House, who was the driving force in letting this book see the light of day; and finally Linda Sewell, whose past faith in Performance Lab began the journey to building all the information in this book. Thanks very much for your effort, faith and support.

APPENDIX

"Troubleshooting" reference section

Remember that most injuries come from training:

→ Too much

→ Too hard

→ Or too different

Other than an "impact" injury most injuries are "overuse" injuries. They will always fall into one of the above three categories AND because they are "overuse" injuries, this immediately implies that in most cases you should be able to detect the overuse before things get too bad and become a problem or injury. The rules of thumb for injuries are usually:

→ While training, if the pain is sharp or intense, stop.

→ If the pain comes on or increases during the run, stop.

→ If you can feel the problem walking around in everyday life, you can't train.

Not rocket science, really, is it?

The great thing about your body is that it let's you know when "overuse" problems begin to build up. You just have to listen carefully enough to respond!

Here are a few common problems and what might be causing them. So why give you this information? While most books focus on how you treat the problem, I think it's better to understand why it is happening so you can stop it before you get to the treatment stage!

Bear in mind that these are not the answers to every problem just more common ones, so please go and see your doctor if you are unsure about how to treat a problem or injury.

Headaches/Breathing feels restricted:

↓ Not relaxing your shoulders and hands

↓ Too much intensity in your training

Suggestion:

↓ Focus on relaxing your shoulders and hands

↓ Think about breathing more deeply (try putting your tongue on the roof of your mouth)

Calf problems:

↓ Too much speed work too soon

↓ Leaning too far forward when you run

↓ Too much uphill running or uphill running at speed (hill is too steep?)

Suggestion:

↓ Try to run more upright (read the information on "balance" in chapter 11)

↓ Cut back on the intensity—buy a heart rate monitor to help you control this! (Most of your running should be at least below 75-80% of maximum heart rate.)

+ Stay off the hills or do them a little slower for a while

Achilles Tendon problems:

+ Too much speed work too soon

+ Leaning too far forward when you run

+ Too much uphill running or uphill running at speed

+ Not enough support around the heel cup of your shoe

+ Too low at the heel or not enough wedge in the shoe (racing flats?)

+ Your shoes are too old

Suggestion:

+ Stay off the hills or do them a little slower for a while

+ Get your shoes looked at by a good running store (the heel cup and wedge)

+ Try to run more upright (read the information on "Balance" in chapter 11)

+ Cut back on the intensity—buy a heart rate monitor to help you control this! (most of your running should be at least below 80% of maximum heart rate)

+ Look at getting several new pairs of shoes (so you always have one pair "worn in" all the time), see chapter 4

Shin problems:

Inside of lower shins

+ Too much speed too soon

+ Running too much on too hard a surface too early

+ Excessive pronation

Epilogue

Suggestion:

+ Slow down (a lot!)

+ See your doctor about treatment if they do not go away in one week or you can feel them when walking around normally

+ Run on softer surfaces

+ Get your shoes looked at by someone experienced at analyzing your running gait

Outside of shins

+ Too fast an increase in training mileage or intensity

Suggestion:

+ See your doctor

+ Back right off, very light running or walking until it goes away

Hip Problems:

Groin — inside of the hip

+ Running hills when tired and running with feet splayed more than usual

+ Too rapid a progression in intensity

+ Favoring another previously injured area

Suggestion:

+ Gentle running if you can't feel your hip or rest until it feels better with some walking

Epilogue

146

↓   Don't run hills when too tired in future

↓   Concentrate on "toes pointing forward" when running hills in future

↓   More progressive ramping of intensity in future

↓   Are you favoring one leg for some reason?

↓   Watch that you don't overstretch this area as you get in and out of cars (particularly, males tend to do this when they're tired and getting into and out of cars that are set up low to the ground).

Outside of the hip behind your hip bone

↓   Too much mileage too soon

Suggestion:

↓   Give yourself a few days to recover

↓   Ramp your mileage slower in future

Knee problems:

Outside of the knee

↓   Tight Iliotibial band which needs stretching

↓   Excessively worn shoes

↓   Running excessively on a sloped road camber

↓   Too much supination

↓   Too much mileage on hard surfaces

Epilogue

↓ Running on very flat road or concrete terrain where footfall is exactly the same each time

Suggestions:

↓ The full name for this problem is Iliotibial Band Friction Syndrome. The band is so tight that it acts like a guitar string on your knee. You need to reduce the friction. Run on gentle mildly uneven, off-road terrain so your footfall is slightly different with each stride so you don't get the friction in the same place all the time.

↓ Get your shoes looked at

↓ Try not to run on the same laterally sloped grade all the time (common from running on gravel roads)

↓ Get your shoes looked at by someone experienced at analyzing your running gait

↓ Ramp your mileage slower in future

↓ Get someone to show you how to stretch your Tensor Fasciae Latae (muscle on the side of your hip)

Inside of the knee

↓ Weak inner quadriceps muscle allowing the knee to drop inward rather than tracking over the second and third toes from the big toe

↓ High Q angle (wider pelvis)

↓ Over pronation

Suggestion:

↓ Concentrate on not letting your knee "drop in" when you run, make sure it tracks over the second and third toe

Epilogue

↓   Get a physical therapist to check the strength balance of your quads and set exercises if needed

↓   Get your shoes looked at by someone experienced at analyzing your running gait

Under or just below the kneecap

↓   Hamstrings are too tight causing foot strike to occur with a more bent knee

↓   Too much downhill running

↓   Too much mileage too soon (particularly on flat, hard roads)

Suggestion:

↓   Stretch hamstrings and quads (see stretching on page 50)

↓   Try to run off road on gentle trails to reduce repetitive inflammation in one area.

↓   Stay off the hills for a while and when you go back try not to run on hills that have long continuous descents

↓   Increase the mileage of your training more slowly

Foot problems:

Black toenails

↓   Shoes don't fit properly or are too wide across the front of the foot

↓   Toenails too long

↓   Long steep downhill running

Epilogue

Suggestion:

+ Get your shoes looked at by a shoe fitting expert

+ Cut your toenails regularly

Pain under the foot between the ball of the foot and heel (Plantar Fasciitis)

+ Flat footed runner

+ No adequate arch support

+ Speed work, hill work or tight calves with little heel support

Suggestion:

+ See a podiatrist

+ Start into your speed work or hill work more gradually in future

+ Make sure you stretch and have flexible calves

Soreness in the balls of the feet

+ Leaning too far forward

+ Running on your toes too much

+ Shoe laces are too tight

Suggestion:

+ Loosen your shoe laces particularly closest to the front of the foot

+ Look at getting a shoe with a wider fit

+ Run more upright (see the information on "Balance" on page 80)

Blisters/chafing

Blisters/chafing on toes or between toes

↓　　　Improper fitting shoes (too small or not wide enough)

Suggestion:

↓　　　Change your shoes to a more appropriate model

↓　　　Tape the area (applying it 12 hours before you run to allow it to cure so it sticks better)

↓　　　Put a lubricant gel (e.g. Vaseline) on the area

↓　　　Buy thicker "breathable" socks

Blisters/chafing just below the ankle on the outside of the foot

↓　　　Not enough gap between the ankle joint and the rim of the shoe

Suggestion:

↓　　　Buy a shoe with a lower rim to allow more ankle freedom (see Chapter 4 on getting the right shoes)

Blisters/chafing on the heel

↓　　　The heel cup does not fit well, allowing your foot to move around in the heel cup excessively

↓　　　There is a ridge in the heel cup where the shoe joins that is rubbing against your heel

Epilogue

Suggestion:

- Buy a new pair of shoes from someone who can analyze your gait and fit your shoes correctly

- Try to "shave off" or cover the vertical ridge seam down the middle of the heel cup

- Buy thicker socks

Blisters/chafing under the front of the foot

- Too much time on the front of your foot (leaning too far forward, running on your toes)

- The width of the shoe is too tight

- Shoe laces are too tight across the front of the foot

- The socks are not breathable enough and the accumulated sweat is causing your foot to get "soft" and blister

Suggestion:

- Buy breathable socks

- Loosen your shoe laces particularly around the front of the foot

- Get a shoe-fitting expert to analyze the best shoe for you

Low back & sciatica problems:

- Poor core stability

- Structural problems caused by degeneration or injury inflamed by running style

- ↓   Too much very steep hill work or speed on hills

- ↓   Rotating your hips excessively forward and back when you run (particularly at speed)

- ↓   Poor hip, hamstring and gluteal flexibility

Suggestion:

- ↓   More core stability training (see a personal trainer)

- ↓   See a doctor for a body/muscle balance examination

- ↓   Stay away from steep hills and speed on hills for a while

- ↓   Try not to rotate your hips excessively when you run (particularly at speed)

Final Notes:

Running off-road on well groomed trails most of the time with some road running, progressing to more road running and, as you get closer to the event, running of the competition distance on the road, will remove the chance of most injuries!

Epilogue

INDEX